Coping with Diabetes in Childhood and Adolescence

Philippa Kaye was educated at Downing College, Cambridge, followed by Guy's, King's and St Thomas's Medical School. Since qualifying as a doctor, she has worked all over London in varying hospital specialities, including general medicine, paediatrics, obstetrics and gynaecology, and psychiatry. She is currently working in general practice in north London. She is the author of *The Fertility Handbook*, also published by Sheldon Press.

Health

Overcoming Common Problems Series

Selected titles

A full list of titles is available from Sheldon Press,
36 Causton Street, London SW1P 4ST and on our website at
www.sheldonpress.co.uk

The Assertiveness Handbook
Mary Hartley

Assertiveness: Step by Step
Dr Windy Dryden and Daniel Constantinou

Body Language: What You Need to Know
David Cohen

Breaking Free
Carolyn Ainscough and Kay Toon

Calm Down
Paul Hauck

The Candida Diet Book
Karen Brody

Cataract: What You Need to Know
Mark Watts

The Chronic Fatigue Healing Diet
Christine Craggs-Hinton

Cider Vinegar
Margaret Hills

Comfort for Depression
Janet Horwood

The Complete Carer's Guide
Bridget McCall

The Confidence Book
Gordon Lamont

Confidence Works
Gladeana McMahon

Coping Successfully with Pain
Neville Shone

Coping Successfully with Panic Attacks
Shirley Trickett

Coping Successfully with Period Problems
Mary-Claire Mason

Coping Successfully with Prostate Cancer
Dr Tom Smith

Coping Successfully with Ulcerative Colitis
Peter Cartwright

Coping Successfully with Your Hiatus Hernia
Dr Tom Smith

Coping Successfully with Your Irritable Bowel
Rosemary Nicol

Coping with Age-related Memory Loss
Dr Tom Smith

Coping with Alopecia
Dr Nigel Hunt and Dr Sue McHale

Coping with Blushing
Dr Robert Edelmann

Coping with Bowel Cancer
Dr Tom Smith

Coping with Brain Injury
Maggie Rich

Coping with Candida
Shirley Trickett

Coping with Chemotherapy
Dr Terry Priestman

Coping with Childhood Allergies
Jill Eckersley

Coping with Childhood Asthma
Jill Eckersley

Coping with Chronic Fatigue
Trudie Chalder

Coping with Coeliac Disease
Karen Brody

Coping with Compulsive Eating
Ruth Searle

Coping with Diverticulitis
Peter Cartwright

Coping with Down's Syndrome
Fiona Marshall

Coping with Dyspraxia
Jill Eckersley

Coping with Eating Disorders and Body Image
Christine Craggs-Hinton

Coping with Endometriosis
Jo Mears

Coping with Family Stress
Dr Peter Cheevers

Overcoming Common Problems Series

Overcoming Common Problems Series

Overcoming Common Problems

Coping with Diabetes in Childhood and Adolescence

DR PHILIPPA KAYE

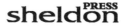
sheldon PRESS

First published in Great Britain in 2008

Sheldon Press
36 Causton Street
London SW1P 4ST

Copyright © Philippa Kaye 2008

British Library Cataloguing-in-Publication Data
A catalogue record for this book is available from the British Library

ISBN 978-1-84709-033-1

1 3 5 7 9 10 8 6 4 2

Typeset by Fakenham Photosetting Ltd, Fakenham, Norfolk
Printed in Great Britain by Ashford Colour Press

Produced on paper from sustainable forests

Contents

Note to the reader

This book is not intended to replace advice from your doctor. If you are concerned regarding your own or your child's health, please contact your local medical services.

Introduction

Most people have heard of diabetes. However, misconceptions abound, from the belief that if you have diabetes you cannot eat anything sweet or nice, to that having diabetes means you will go blind. Thankfully, these ideas are not entirely correct! Having a child diagnosed with a lifelong, currently incurable condition such as diabetes, or being diagnosed with one yourself, is daunting. Some people respond by voraciously reading everything they can about the subject, from articles in the press to medical books and searching the internet; others do not. Everyone will have different reactions, such as bewilderment, anger, and the common, 'Why me?' You may be offered counselling to help you through this potentially difficult period.

Diabetes is a common condition in which the body either cannot produce or cannot respond to insulin, a hormone used by cells so they can use the glucose we obtain from our food to make energy. There are various types of diabetes: the commonest in childhood is type 1 diabetes, when the body stops producing insulin, which then has to be replaced via insulin injections. If there is no insulin, the cells of the body cannot access the glucose in the bloodstream, which can cause both short-term and long-term complications.

Parents take a lot of the responsibility for their child's health. Doctors and nurses can give advice and offer treatments but, as with all medical care, you will decide how much of this you accept. Initially this can be overwhelming; you may feel you have a lot to learn and that your entire life is changing. With time, however, looking after your child's diabetes simply becomes part of everyday life. In fact, you will go from not knowing very much about diabetes to being the expert, and you will find yourself teaching other people, such as teachers, friends and babysitters about diabetes. You will be given as much help as you need along the way from the doctors, nurses, dieticians and counsellors who make up your diabetes team.

The aim of this book is to help you gain some understanding about diabetes. Topics covered include how the body absorbs food, what diabetes actually is, its monitoring and treatments, a healthy diet and how to manage and prevent emergencies and long-term complications. Although the book can be read straight through, some parts may not be relevant to you at certain stages. For example, if you have a child diagnosed with diabetes at the age of four, you do not need to read the section on diabetes and puberty just yet! Conversely, if you are diagnosed with diabetes in your teens, this book can be read by both you and your parents. You can dip into the book when new situations occur, such as going to a birthday party, staying up all night, or if a child becomes unwell. Throughout the book there are boxes of common questions that can be used for quick reference when needed. Different people learn in different ways and no book can ever replace a trip to see your diabetes team. If at any point, in any situation, you feel that you cannot manage, contact your team for advice.

Diabetes involves the whole family and not just the child affected. Although initially it may feel like it, diabetes will not run your and your family's lives. It simply becomes part of everyday life; eating well, monitoring and giving injections will become as ordinary as going to school, doing homework or household chores. It is the aim of this book to help with the process of making your diabetes ordinary. You control and manage your diabetes and not the other way around!

Terms used in this book. The terms blood glucose and blood sugar levels are used interchangeably. Blood contains plasma and various blood cells. The terms blood glucose or blood sugar are used here to describe the level of glucose that can be found in the plasma. Blood glucose levels are described in the units mmol/l, that is, how much glucose is in one litre of blood, even though only a very small drop is tested. You may find that in other countries or books, the units used to describe blood glucose levels are different. Hyperglycaemia means the levels of plasma glucose are high, hypoglycaemia, that they are low.

1

The control of blood glucose and diabetes

In order to fully understand and therefore take control of your child's diabetes you need an understanding of how the body absorbs glucose (sugar) from food, why glucose is needed and how the body controls blood sugar levels.

Why do you need glucose?

The body is made up of different organs and structures, which in turn are made of millions and millions of tiny cells. For these cells to live and function a supply of both glucose and oxygen is needed. The cells convert the glucose and oxygen into energy, carbon dioxide and water. The energy produced is used to make the cells work so the body can function. The process by which the cells convert the glucose into energy is known as respiration. The oxygen is obtained from the air we breathe in, we then breathe out the carbon dioxide produced.

Where do you get glucose from?

Our food can be divided into three main groups: starches and sugars; protein and fat. Most of this chapter focuses on starches and sugars. The body breaks down proteins such as meat, fish or nuts into their smallest parts, amino acids, which are then used to make up the different cells and tissues of the body. The fat is broken down into tiny droplets and used to help build the body's nervous system including nerves and the brain. Fat can also be used to store energy for use later.

The body gets its glucose from food. Glucose is a form of sugar, but you don't just get it from eating sugary sweets. We get starches and sugars from any carbohydrates we eat such as potatoes and pasta. The body breaks down these starches into sugar molecules. From healthy complex carbohydrates such as rice and oats to more refined carbohydrates like those found in cakes and biscuits, all carbohydrates are eventually broken down into glucose. The difference between the complex and refined carbohydrates is how quickly they are converted to glucose. There are different types of sugar such as simple sugars, glucose and fructose; the different types are converted into glucose for use in the body.

How does the body absorb glucose?

The digestive system begins to break down carbohydrates as soon as you put them in your mouth. Your saliva contains an enzyme called amylase that breaks down carbohydrate into long chains of sugars. When you swallow, the food passes through a tube called the oesophagus into your stomach. In the stomach the food is mixed with stomach acid to help break it down further.

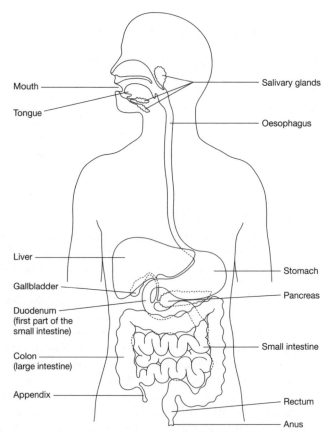

Figure 1 The anatomy of the digestive system

Food can be held in the stomach for a short time. The stomach releases a bit of the food at a time into the small intestine (see Figure 1). The body produces other enzymes from the pancreas which are then released into the small intestine and break the food up even further, after which the complex carbohydrate of the potato you ate is now a simple glucose molecule. The more complex the carbohydrate, the longer it takes to be broken down, so granary bread takes a lot longer than a chocolate biscuit.

Once the carbohydrate is broken up into glucose and other sugars it can be absorbed into the body. Therefore this only happens once the food has got to the small intestine, from which the sugars are absorbed into the bloodstream. So, the faster the food can be broken down, the faster it can cause a rise in blood sugar levels. Quick rises are often followed by significant drops in blood glucose levels, and these drops can affect the body. Among other things they may make you feel tired and hungry. If a food is broken down more slowly, it gives a slower prolonged release of sugar into the bloodstream, so blood sugar levels do not peak and fall so rapidly. Therefore, sweets and white bread get into the bloodstream quickly to bring up your blood sugar if needed, but more complex foods such as porridge help give a steady release of sugar and therefore energy over a longer period of time without the peaks and falls in blood sugar levels.

Where does the body store glucose?

The circulation of the body is wired so that the blood coming from the small intestine, full of glucose, reaches the liver before any other structure. Much of the glucose is absorbed by the liver and converted into glycogen. Glycogen can then be converted back into glucose when the body needs it. Glycogen can be considered a glucose store. When you have a lot of glucose in the blood, the body creates glycogen; when levels are low such as at night or during starvation the body uses up its glycogen stores to ensure that the cells continue to get glucose to produce energy and therefore function correctly. The liver cannot store enough glucose in the form of glycogen to last very long. It can store enough glucose to last a child approximately 12 hours without food, a baby much less time and an adult for 24 hours.

The glucose left in the blood then passes to the rest of the body for use by all the cells in the production of energy. Your muscles can also store glucose as glycogen. However, unlike the glycogen stores of the liver, which can be used in times of need by the rest of the body, the glycogen stores of muscles can only be used by the muscles during exercise.

What happens after a meal?

Let's assume that you eat three meals a day – forget about snacks for the moment to keep things simple. During and after a meal your body uses sugars absorbed directly into the bloodstream from the small intestine for energy and to rebuild the stores of glycogen. About four hours after you finish a meal, there is probably not much sugar left to be absorbed from the small intestine and so the levels of sugar within the blood begin to fall. At this point the liver stores of glycogen can be broken down to be used as glucose by the body. Eventually, probably about six hours after your last meal, you eat again, the cycle restarts and the stores of glycogen can be reformed.

If you eat snacks between meals, your blood sugar levels rise and you may not need to use your glycogen stores. However, excess glucose can be stored as fat, so eating more than you need causes you to put on weight.

How does the body control the level of glucose in the blood?

Blood glucose levels are controlled by a complicated system of different hormones. Hormones are substances produced in one part of the body that allow something to happen in another part of the body, for example allowing cells to use glucose. The main hormones involved in the control of blood glucose are produced by the pancreas. The pancreas is an organ that sits just under your stomach; it produces insulin and other enzymes to help digest your food. The pancreas is made up of many smaller structures called islets of Langerhans – within these, certain cells (beta cells) produce insulin and others (alpha cells) produce glucagon, two important hormones in the control of blood sugar. These substances are released from the pancreas into the small intestine. The explanation below refers to the situation within a person without diabetes.

What does insulin do and how does it work?

Insulin allows cells to use the glucose in the blood, and therefore has the effect of lowering blood glucose levels.

Insulin allows cells to use glucose in the blood in the production of energy. It sticks to the surface of the cells and acts like a gatekeeper to allow glucose to enter the cell. Insulin also stops the liver from releasing glucose from its stores of glycogen; in fact it stimulates the liver to use the glucose for storage in glycogen for use in the future. Insulin has other functions such as stimulating the production of protein in the body; if you eat more than you need, insulin stimulates the excess carbohydrate to be turned into fat. In times of starvation, these fat stores can be broken back down to glucose to release energy and ketones.

When you eat a meal, the beta cells in the pancreas detect the rise in blood sugar and start to release insulin. They only secrete the correct amount of insulin needed according to the amount of food eaten. This happens very quickly, so in someone without diabetes there should not be a large rise in blood sugar volumes after a meal. Even when you are not eating, for example at night, your body is still releasing glucose from your stores in the liver. Therefore the pancreas still needs to release insulin, though in a much smaller amount, so cells can use the glucose that is being produced. This is called the 'basal insulin'. Nearly half of the insulin produced per day is from this background secretion of insulin. During and after mealtimes much more insulin is produced, and these peaks of insulin are called the 'bolus insulin'.

What is glucagon and how does it work?

Glucagon can almost be considered the opposite of insulin as it acts to increase the amount of glucose within the blood. Glucagon is produced by the alpha cells of the islets of Langerhans in the pancreas and is released when blood sugars are falling or low, as occurs during the night. It acts by stimulating the liver to release glucose from its stores of glycogen and also stimulates the breakdown of fat and proteins to produce further glucose.

Other hormones are also involved in blood sugar control. Adrenaline, growth hormone and the stress hormone cortisol all increase the level of sugar within the blood.

The 'balancing act'

You can consider the control of blood glucose levels to be a balancing act or tightrope (see Figure 2, overleaf). On the one hand are situations and substances that increase blood sugar, and on the other are situations and substances that decrease blood glucose levels. It is very important

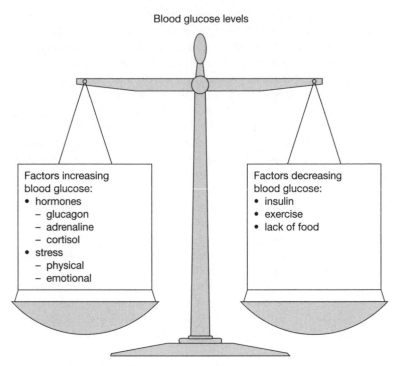

Figure 2 **The balancing act of blood glucose control**

that the balance is correct, as both too little and too much are potentially dangerous. The body uses the hormones described above to keep blood glucose levels between about 4 and 7 mmol/l. The medical term for blood sugars within the normal range is 'normoglycaemia', for blood sugars which are high, 'hyperglycaemia', and for blood sugars which are low, 'hypoglycaemia'. These terms are used throughout the book.

When sugars are reaching the upper limit of normal or even higher, the pancreas produces insulin to bring them back down. When the levels are reaching the lower limit of normal, the pancreas produces glucagon and the rest of the body produces the other hormones mentioned above such as adrenaline to bring the levels back up to normal. Other factors are involved in the balancing act; obviously food brings up the blood glucose, as does stress. Exercise and not eating lower the blood glucose. All these factors interplay together to keep the body's glucose level tightly within the normal range.

It might seem strange that only one hormone lowers blood glucose, while many increase the levels. This is because even at a slightly lower level than normal – for example even at a blood sugar level of 3.5 mmol/l – you begin to feel unwell and every system in the body is affected. The brain cannot store glucose as the liver can, and so relies on glucose that it can absorb from the bloodstream. So the body must act defensively to increase the level of glucose so that the brain is working properly. This is called 'counter-regulation'.

During prolonged periods of low glucose levels or even starvation, the hormones release glucose from the stores within the liver (glyco-genolysis) and also produce glucose from fat stores (gluconeogenesis). As described above, the blood from the small intestine which is full of glucose from your last meal, combined with insulin, first goes to the liver for storage. An adult can store about 100g of glucose in the liver, a child much less, though the average 5-year-old has enough stores to manage about 12 hours without affecting blood sugar, as happens at night. The younger the child, the smaller the stores of glycogen. It is important to note that even if a young child is not active she uses up glucose much quicker than an adult.

Other factors affect levels apart from eating, exercise and insulin.

Growth hormone is one of the hormones that increases blood glucose. That is not its only role – as its name suggests, it is needed for growth. Therefore, in teenagers who are growing a lot, the increased amount of growth hormone produced leads to a rise in blood glucose so more insulin must be secreted to balance this.

Adrenaline, the hormone of 'fright, fight or flight', is produced in all stressful situations. Historically and in terms of evolution, a 'fright' would mean being attacked by something and the only options would be to respond ('fight') or to run away ('flight'); both of these need increased amounts of glucose, so adrenaline also increases blood glucose. Today, 'fright' describes any stressful situation from an exam, an argument, playing computer games or even being ill. As adrenaline is produced, among its many actions is an increase in blood sugar. More insulin is produced to balance this and keep glucose levels within normal range.

Ketones

As described above, the body can produce glucose and therefore energy from the breakdown of its stores of fat. A by-product of this fat break-down are ketones, which can be used as fuel by some parts of the body such as the brain.

The body starts to break down fat when it cannot access glucose.

This can be during starvation when the glycogen stores have run out, but also in diabetes. In diabetes, there is plenty of glucose in the blood, but the cells cannot access it without the gatekeeper insulin. So the body acts as if it is starving and starts to break down fat and produce ketones. Ketones can lead to symptoms such as vomiting, and unless treated can become dangerous. (See Chapter 7 on diabetic emergencies.) Hopefully, you now have some understanding of how and why the body uses and regulates blood glucose levels, which will help you understand diabetes and its treatment.

What is diabetes?

Diabetes, short for diabetes mellitus, is a condition in which the levels of glucose in the blood are higher than normal. The hormonal control of blood glucose is not working as it should. Diabetes comes from the Greek word *diabainein*, in its meaning 'to siphon' or 'pass through', referring to a flow of liquid. The condition was named by a second-century Greek physician Aretaeus the Cappadocian, to describe one of the major symptoms of diabetes – increased and frequent urination, i.e. they urinated like a siphon! The word 'mellitus' was added in the seventeenth century and is from the Latin word for honey (*mel*) when it was noted that those with diabetes passed urine with a sweet taste (due to the excess glucose).

The term diabetes as used in this book refers only to diabetes mellitus and its subtypes. The condition diabetes insipidus also involves frequent urination but in this condition insulin and blood glucose levels are normal. Diabetes mellitus used to be divided into two subgroups, 'insulin dependent diabetes mellitus (IDDM)' and 'non-insulin dependent diabetes mellitus (NIDDM)'. This classification is now rarely used.

Subtypes of diabetes

Type 1 diabetes

Type 1 diabetes is an autoimmune disease, a condition in which the body attacks itself. The insulin-producing cells of the pancreas are attacked by the body so that insulin is no longer produced. Initially only some of the cells are destroyed so some insulin continues to be produced, but with time the production of insulin falls and eventually the pancreas no longer produces insulin.

What happens when no insulin is produced?

Glucose is still absorbed from food, but without insulin it cannot get into the cells, resulting in high levels of glucose within the blood. Some of this excess glucose is passed out of the body via the kidneys and urine, resulting in the sweet urine that gives diabetes its name.

As the cells cannot obtain glucose from the blood without insulin, they act as if the body is in starvation mode. Although there is plenty of glucose in the blood, the cells cannot use it and so give signals to the body that blood sugar is low. Hormones that increase blood glucose, such as glucagon, are secreted, resulting in the release of glucose from the stores of glycogen in the liver, further driving up the blood glucose. Despite this, as no insulin is being produced, the cells still cannot access the glucose in the blood. They continue to respond as if starvation is occurring and so fat stores are broken down into two parts – fatty acids and glycerol. The glycerol is then further broken down into glucose and the fatty acids into ketones. At this point there are high levels of both glucose and ketones in the bloodstream, both of which are excreted in the urine.

Type 1 diabetes is insulin dependent – that is, it can only be treated with insulin. Once insulin is given, it acts as the gatekeeper just as the body's natural production of insulin does, allowing the cells to access the glucose in the bloodstream and encouraging the production of glycogen stores in the liver, bringing blood glucose levels back to normal.

In a nutshell, the body does not realize that it has diabetes: all it responds to is the fact that the cells do not have access to glucose. Therefore it tries to increase the amount of glucose in the blood and eventually goes into starvation mode. The high levels of blood glucose are potentially very harmful, though this can be corrected with insulin. Type 1 diabetes is the commonest type of diabetes in childhood. Over 90 per cent of children with diabetes have type 1.

Type 2 diabetes

In type 2 diabetes some insulin is still produced by the pancreas. However, either not enough insulin is produced, or the body cannot respond to the insulin, and it becomes increasingly less sensitive to the insulin produced – 'insulin resistance'. As the cells are less responsive blood glucose levels remain high, so the pancreas produces more insulin to try and control this. Eventually, as the pancreas becomes exhausted, production may stop altogether. With time, as the body becomes increasingly less able to respond to the insulin produced, the cells respond as in the situation described for type 1 diabetes above.

Type 2 diabetes used to be thought of as a condition that only occurred in adults. However, the incidence of type 2 diabetes in children is increasing. This may be because type 2 diabetes is associated with being overweight and the number of overweight children has also increased.

Type 2 diabetes can initially be controlled using diet and lifestyle changes. Oral medication can also be used. These medications cannot increase the amount of insulin produced. Rather, they increase the sensitivity of the cells to the insulin that the pancreas is already secreting. In some people, treatment with insulin may still be needed.

Maturity onset diabetes of the young

Maturity onset diabetes of the young (MODY) is a rare genetic, inherited form of diabetes that can be treated with diet, tablets or insulin. Due to its rarity, it will not be discussed further in this book.

Latent autoimmune diabetes in the adult

Latent autoimmune diabetes in the adult is a subtype of type 1 diabetes. Here, the body is very sensitive to insulin and therefore can cope with the decreasing amount of insulin produced so may not develop symptoms until a later age.

How common is diabetes?

According to the International Diabetes Federation, worldwide it is estimated that over 400,000 children aged 14 and under have diabetes. This number is thought to be rising. The number of people with diabetes varies between different countries, e.g. diabetes is much more common in Scandinavia than in Japan for reasons as yet unknown. Diabetes is one of the commonest chronic conditions of childhood. For all children affected, over 90 per cent have type 1 diabetes.

In England and Wales about 15 per 100,000 children develop diabetes each year. It is more common in Scotland with about 25 per 100,000 children developing the condition. The number of children with diabetes is significantly higher now than 50 years ago and the incidence is thought to be rising.

As mentioned above, type 1 diabetes is thought to be an autoimmune condition, where the body attacks itself. There are some markers which can be tested for by blood tests for autoimmunity and many children with diabetes will be positive. However, these markers can be present in those without diabetes, who never go on to develop the condition, and so cannot be used to predict who will and who will not develop diabetes.

Why do you get diabetes?

At present, scientists and doctors do not know what exactly causes diabetes, though various explanations have been suggested.

Possible causes of type 1 diabetes

Infectious disease

It is possible that a virus triggers off the autoimmune process that results in the destruction of the insulin consistency producing beta cells in the pancreas. It may do this by being very similar in structure to one of the proteins in the beta cells, so the body's defence system cannot tell the difference between the virus it wants to destroy and the cells it wants to keep. It may be that repeated attacks of the virus are needed to cause diabetes.

The 'hygiene hypothesis'

Children now get many fewer infections than in the past, due to improved standards of hygiene. It is possible that this has resulted in their immune systems reacting differently when they do meet infections. Infections immediately after birth appear to increase the risk of diabetes, perhaps as the immune system is immature.

Genetic predisposition

However, only approximately 10 per cent of children with diabetes have a parent or sibling with the condition.

Maternal infection

If a mother develops certain infections during pregnancy such as rubella (German measles), there is an increased risk of the child developing diabetes.

Environmental factors

For example, it is more common to develop diabetes in the winter due to a need for increased insulin production.

Early exposure to cow's milk

At less than six months, for example, this may be a factor, as in countries where children do not drink milk there is less childhood diabetes.

This is not a proven theory, and while cow's milk is not recommended in those under six months, after this age milk is encouraged as a healthy food and good source of calcium.

Possible causes of type 2 diabetes

Genetic predisposition

The likelihood of inheriting a predisposition to type 2 diabetes appears to be much stronger than inheriting a predisposition to type 1. Many of those with type 2 diabetes have a parent or family history of the condition; the numbers quoted range from 25 per cent to as high as 80 per cent.

Obesity

Being overweight increases the likelihood of developing type 2 diabetes. About 80 per cent of people with type 2 diabetes are overweight. It may be that a predisposition to being overweight may be inherited from your parents. Extra fat in the cells makes it harder for them to respond to insulin.

Ethnicity

Certain ethnic groups such as Asian or African people are more likely to develop type 2 diabetes.

For both type 1 and type 2 diabetes it is most likely that a combination of factors results in the condition.

Why is diabetes important?

It is important to try and maintain blood glucose within normal levels in order for the body to function properly. Both too high and too low levels are emergencies and can be very dangerous, and there are potential long-term complications of the condition (see Chapters 7 and 8 for further information).

Common questions

- *Can you catch diabetes?* No. It is important that your child and her friends, teachers and parents know that diabetes is not infectious, as this may not be obvious to them. Simple education helps your child to be accepted by her peers.

- *Can you be tested to see if you are going to get diabetes?* At present, this is not possible. Children with diabetes do carry some markers in their blood, but the same marker is carried by lots of children who do not develop diabetes and so it cannot be used as a predictive test.
- *Can diabetes be prevented?* Unfortunately at present, type 1 diabetes cannot be prevented. However, lifestyle adjustments, good diet and treatment can help prevent long-term complications. As type 2 diabetes is thought to be related to being overweight, controlling weight may be preventative.
- *Can you get diabetes from eating too many sweets or sugary foods?* Not type 1 diabetes. It is a common misbelief, as once a person has diabetes, he or she tends to stop eating sugary foods. With type 2 diabetes, eating sweets specifically does not cause the condition; rather it is related to being overweight. Therefore a diet with an excess of calories, such as one rich in sugary foods, can lead to obesity and an increased risk of type 2 diabetes.
- *If my child is overweight, will he definitely get diabetes?* Not definitely, but he is at increased risk of type 2 diabetes.
- *Is it my fault that my child got diabetes?* Definitely not. Type 1 diabetes is no one's 'fault', it is a condition that happens, for reasons as yet not really known, that currently cannot be prevented. There is no need to blame yourself. A healthy diet and physical exercise help decrease the risk of type 2 diabetes, so this is one area where you can take action.

2

Finding out that it's diabetes

Finding out that your child has diabetes can be a difficult time. Hearing that your child is unwell is hard enough; learning that he has a chronic condition, and having to learn about its management is hugely daunting, though you should have lots of help from your local diabetes team and GP (see below). Do talk to the nurses, doctors, friends, partners and, most importantly, your child.

Symptoms and signs of type 1 diabetes

Diabetes symptoms can sometimes be recognized at an early stage. However, diabetes is often not picked up until the child is unwell and may require a stay in hospital. The most frequent and 'classic' symptoms of type 1 diabetes are:

- increased thirst (polydypsia) – drinking lots more than usual;
- increased urination (polyuria) – needing and going to the toilet to pass urine more frequently than usual, especially at night. This is sometimes seen as an increase in the number of wetting accidents a child has (either in the day or at night);
- weight loss;
- tired all the time.

Other symptoms that are common in children include:

- abdominal pain – tummy aches and other tummy problems;
- headaches;
- problems with behaviour such as problems with concentration, or naughtiness.

The condition may develop over a few weeks, so you may notice the above symptoms. Alternatively if your child develops tummy-aches or any illness that is unexplained, or does not really get better, she should have her blood sugar levels tested. Diabetes can often come on so rapidly that it is not possible to pick up any symptoms before a child becomes unwell. The child may develop ketoacidosis (see Chapter 7, 'Diabetic emergencies'), requiring hospital admission and treatment. Diabetes can be diagnosed at any age.

Symptoms and signs of type 2 diabetes

The symptoms and signs of type 2 diabetes can be the same as for type 1, though very often there are no symptoms at all. Type 2 diabetes is often picked up when someone is unwell or being tested for other conditions. However, given that being overweight is a risk factor for type 2 diabetes, if either you or your child is overweight keep a close eye for the above symptoms, or if you are worried at all ask for a blood sugar test at your GP.

How is diabetes diagnosed?

Diabetes is diagnosed by blood tests that measure the level of glucose in the blood. Normally blood glucose levels lie between about 4 and 6 mmol/l. The blood test can be taken after a six-hour fast, generally first thing in the morning, or at a random time of the day. Fasting samples are considered much more accurate.

Diabetes can be diagnosed if:

- a fasting venous blood glucose level is over 7.0 mmol/l;
- a random venous blood glucose level is over 11.1 mmol/l.

A further test is called the oral glucose tolerance test. Here a fasting blood sample is taken, generally first thing in the morning after a six-hour fast. You then drink a drink that contains 75 g of glucose (often in the form of a certain amount of Lucozade) and wait two hours. After two hours a second blood sample is taken. The results are analysed according to Table 1.

The table includes a column called 'impaired glucose tolerance'; this does not mean that you have diabetes but that you are at increased risk of developing type 2 diabetes. Children who are unwell with one high blood glucose test can be diagnosed with diabetes.

You may find that your doctor may screen your child for dia-

Table 1 Analyses of blood glucose levels

Blood glucose level (mmol/l)	Normal	Impaired glucose tolerance	Diabetes mellitus
Fasting sample (after a 6-hour fast)	4–6	Above 6 but less than 7.0	Above 7.0
Random sample (2 hours after 75 g glucose load)	Less than 7.0	Between 7.0 and 11.1	Above 11.1

betes using a finger-prick test or a urine test (discussed in Chapter 3, 'Monitoring diabetes'). Diabetes cannot be diagnosed from these tests alone; a fasting blood sample is required.

What happens now?

The explanation below refers to type 1 diabetes; type 2 diabetes is generally managed at home, with outpatient appointments, as discussed later (see Chapter 5, 'Treatment of diabetes').

What happens once diabetes is diagnosed depends on how well or unwell your child is at the time and on your local medical services. Type 1 diabetes is *always* treated with insulin injections; it simply cannot be treated with oral medicines. So in the first days and weeks after diagnosis you will learn among many other things how to give the injections, monitor blood glucose levels, and about a healthy diet.

If your child is well, you may have the option of starting treatment at home, depending on the resources of the diabetic team in your area. Even if your child is well the amount of insulin he needs changes regularly, even daily, especially at the beginning of treatment. This may well appear daunting but you will be given the phone number of someone in the diabetes team whom you can contact at any time. It is really important that you do ask those questions and the team should encourage you to do so!

Not all areas can provide a service that allows you to start treatment at home with the continuous support of the diabetes team. In some areas, even if your child is well, you may be asked to come into hospital for a short period to start treatment. Even if you are offered home treatment you may prefer to start treatment in hospital as this may make you feel more secure while you are learning – please tell your doctor if this is the case.

If your child is unwell you will be asked to start treatment in hospital. If your child presents with ketoacidosis the initial treatment is more aggressive, with an intravenous line to give fluids and insulin directly into the body.

Help!

Of course, this is a scary time, not just for your child but also for you and your family. As a parent you may be faced with the situation where your child cries or fights you about having an injection, and some people have a phobia of needles. It is always difficult to be told that your child is unwell, and in this case has a chronic condition. The doctors, nurses and other members of the team understand this and are there as people to talk to. You may also ask for counselling if you feel you would benefit from someone else to talk to about your experiences. It is important to keep talking and asking as many questions as you need. No question is too simple and no one will think you are stupid if you keep asking and repeating the same questions. Now is the time to ask those questions and to learn the basics so that you can manage diabetes to the best of your ability.

It is common to blame yourself or start asking why this has happened. It is not your fault and we do not know why diabetes occurs. If it all seems too much for you then speak out and say so; you will get the support and help you need.

Diabetes is a chronic condition, and yes, as yet there is no cure; however, diabetes can be controlled very well. It does not mean that your child will not have a 'normal life'. He will be able to do whatever he wants, he will just also have to manage his diabetes at the same time. Unbelievable as it may sound at the beginning, with time, caring for your diabetes, calculating how much insulin is needed, giving injections and eating a healthy diet will become manageable, ordinary and just part of daily life.

The first few weeks

Once insulin is given and blood sugar levels begin to return to normal, you may find that your child begins to feel better very quickly. He may also become very hungry, especially if he has recently lost weight. The amount of insulin is adjusted according to how much he eats. Within a few weeks your child will be back to eating normally.

Your diabetes team

The team works closely together and generally includes a paediatrician often specializing in or with an interest in diabetes, a diabetes specialist nurse, other nurses, a dietician and often a child psychologist and/or a counsellor. These people make up your multidisciplinary team, and others may be involved if needed, for example a kidney doctor if your child develops kidney problems etc.

The doctor and nurses work out the starting doses of insulin and show you how to give injections, what emergency symptoms and signs to look out for, how to calculate the doses of insulin each day, and what to do when your child is unwell. The dietician gives advice regarding a healthy diet and may again help you calculate the doses of insulin required with each meal. The psychologist and/or counsellor may help you with telling your child, managing your child's response, and also look after you. You are part of this team and as such your contribution is valid and encouraged. You can draw on the support and skills of the team to help you through this period of adjustment and during the future. The team has many roles, not simply the medical care of diabetes, but also support, counselling, family support and education and liaison with other organizations, such as schools.

If you have a partner, then it is important that both of you are educated about diabetes – matters such as changes in the household diet, warning symptoms and emergency treatment. If you do not have a partner then you may have another person such as a close friend or parent to confide in, or indeed anyone on the diabetes team.

The age of your child determines what and how much he is told about his condition. Obviously if the child is very young, the majority of the education is directed at parents. However, children are encouraged to learn about and take some control over their diabetes from an early age so that they can begin to take responsibility for their own condition.

Topics that will be discussed with your team after diabetes is diagnosed

- what diabetes is
- how to monitor blood glucose levels
- the symptoms of low and high blood glucose levels
- what equipment is needed and how to use it
- how to give insulin injections
- what to do for hypoglycaemia and hyperglycaemia
- healthy diet
- what to tell school/family/friends.

3

Monitoring diabetes

It is important to monitor glucose levels regularly. This chapter focuses on how to monitor diabetes in both the short and long term. The tests to monitor diabetes are the same for both type 1 and type 2. However, the frequency of testing may differ depending on your diagnosis and treatment. Your diabetes team can advise you on what is appropriate.

Finger-prick blood tests

This tells you the level of glucose in the blood at the precise moment the test is taken. Therefore these results can change quite quickly. Information about blood glucose levels can be used, for example, to calculate how much insulin is needed before a meal, or if someone is feeling unwell it can tell if she is hypo- or hyperglycaemic.

How do I take a finger prick?

First wash your hands and those of your child – this is to wash off any sugar that might be on your hands and give an incorrect reading, and also for hygiene reasons to prevent infection. Use warm water to increase the blood flow to the fingers to make it easier to obtain a drop of blood.

You should have been given a finger-pricking device and a small machine that calculate the glucose levels. You will be shown how to take a finger prick, as different machines work in different ways. Many devices are loaded with springs, you load the lancet (cutting device) into a machine and then hold the machine against the skin and press a button, the lancet pops out and pierces the skin. Most people find these machines easy and safe to use. A drop of blood is taken and then put in the machine to calculate blood glucose. This can be momentarily painful.

Prick the side of the finger after the last joint, near the fingertip. Pricking the side of the fingertip instead of the pad of the finger is less painful and also has less effect on the sensitivity of the finger itself. Try to avoid pricking your thumbs and index finger of the dominant hand (i.e. right hand in right-handed people) as these are used most for sensation.

Some machines store the readings for a few days or weeks, otherwise you can write them down in a diary or transfer them to your computer to get a good idea of the pattern of glucose readings and therefore the control of your child's diabetes.

How often should I take a finger-prick test?

Your doctor will advise you how often to take blood tests. The tests are taken so that you can act on the results and adjust the insulin dose accordingly. In type 1 diabetes, it is thought that at least four tests are necessary each day so that your child can take the correct dose of insulin. These four tests should be before breakfast, lunch and dinner and before going to bed.

Some doctors recommend that you take a full 24-hour glucose profile at least once a fortnight. This means that you take finger-prick tests before and two hours after every meal, and once during the night.

There are times when you may need to take more than four tests per day, for example when going out for a late meal or a party and eating differently to normal, when exercising a lot, when unwell, as with a cold, or during emotional stress. In these situations, insulin require-ments may be different to normal and so it is appropriate to take a test before and two hours after each meal so that you can adjust the dose of insulin.

Tests can also be taken when your child feels unwell to help you recognize a hypoglycaemic reaction.

What should the value be?

The target is to have a blood glucose level between 4 and 7 or 8 mmol/l before meals (pre-prandial) and up to 10 mmol/l, but preferably no higher, two hours after you eat a meal (post-prandial). If your levels are higher or lower than these, insulin treatment may need adjusting.

It is helpful if you can keep a diary or logbook of your readings. Also note if your child is doing lots of physical activity, or eating differently from normal (older children and teenagers may want to do this them-selves). A diary is very useful so that both you and your diabetes team can monitor your treatment and see if the doses need changing.

Is the reading correct?

No machine is perfect, and each has a different margin of error, which should be detailed in the information given with the machine. For example, if the margin of error is 10 per cent, a blood sugar level of 10 mmol/l can actually be between 9 and 11 mmol/l; however, a low blood sugar reading of 2 can only be between 1.8 and 2.2 mmol/l. Therefore the machines are more accurate at lower blood glucose readings.

In order to get a true reading, you must use the machine correctly. Incorrectly high readings may be because there was glucose on the fingers (the reason why you should wash your hands before testing). Incorrectly low readings may be because the drop of blood put on the strip was too small.

If the machine says 'low' or 'high', do not presume that this is an incorrect reading. It may mean that the levels are too high or too low to be picked up by the machine. These readings should be acted on as soon as possible.

Common questions

- *Does pricking the fingers cause a loss of sensation?* The skin may become thicker over time but there is currently no evidence that shows a significant loss of sensation over time. Pricking on the side of the fingers is less painful than the pads, but also means that even if there is some loss of sensation it should not affect function.
- *Do I have to use the fingers?* No, fingers are easiest to get to but you could use toes as long as the feet are healthy. If there are problems with wounds or decreased sensation on the feet you must not use your toes. Alternative machines may sample different places such as the thigh but these are considered less accurate.
- *My child cries and struggles when I try to finger-prick him: what should I do?* This is a difficult situation; he may be scared, or it hurts or he simply doesn't want to do it – distressing for both him and you. If you need to, ask someone else to hold him tightly, so that he cannot move his arms and struggle. Although it sounds horrible, this means that you can do the test as quickly as possible to minimize the stress for all concerned. Then give your child a cuddle and try and comfort him. He may try to reject you, but try to explain why you are doing it and that getting the test out of the way quickly is the best thing to do.
- *How can I make it hurt less?* Try rubbing the finger with an ice cube to anaesthetize it before taking the test.
- *My child says she is scared of the blood: how can I help?* Emphasize the importance of the test in keeping her well. Ask her what it is

that scares her – is it the needle, or the blood itself? She may be scared that she will run out of blood, in which case reassure her that the body makes more all the time, so one little drop won't make a difference. Try doing the test on yourself to show there is nothing to be scared of.

- *What should the values be?* Between about 4 and 7 mmol/l before a meal and up to 10 mmol/l two hours after a meal.
- *My child's levels are always higher than the recommended values: what should I do?* Speak to your team – the doses of insulin may need changing. With time you may become confident enough to make such changes yourself.

Urine tests

Urine glucose

Urine tests used to be the only method of diagnosing diabetes. Before the advent of blood tests and blood glucose monitoring, doctors would diagnose diabetes by smelling and often tasting the urine for sweetness. Urine tests are useful, but not as accurate as finger-prick tests.

Your kidneys produce urine from the water and waste products of your body. Therefore, whatever is found in the urine can reflect what is in the body. The kidneys try to reabsorb as much glucose from the blood as they can. Once blood glucose levels are too high for the kidneys to reabsorb all the glucose, the rest is passed out in the urine. The level at which the kidneys cannot reabsorb any more glucose is called the renal threshold. The average renal threshold corresponds to a blood glucose level, on average between 8 and 10 mmol/l in children.

You can consider that the amount of glucose in the urine reflects the amount of glucose in the blood since the last time you went to the toilet. While blood glucose testing shows the current levels, urine glucose testing shows the level over the previous few hours. Even if you take the blood glucose level before each meal, the glucose can still go up in between these times. Taking a urine glucose test tells you if this is occurring.

Urine glucose tests are less accurate than blood glucose tests, especially if you have a much higher or lower than average renal threshold for glucose – that is, you excrete glucose in your urine at a higher or lower level than normal. Your diabetes team can show you how to calculate the renal glucose threshold. Urine glucose tests can be useful if for some reason you cannot test your blood sugar.

Urine ketones

High levels of urinary ketones, excreted in the urine, imply very low levels of insulin and potentially dangerously high blood glucose levels.

How do you test urine for glucose and ketones?

Most urine tests rely on a 'dipstick' system. Your child wees into a pot or the potty; with children in nappies, you can very often squeeze a drop or two of urine from the nappy. You will be given a box of urine dipstick test strips to use and shown how to use them by your diabetes team.

The dipstick looks like a thin strip of paper with raised small coloured squares on it, each square representing a substance potentially found in the urine, such as glucose or ketones (see Figure 3). You dip the dipstick into the urine and wait; after a set amount of time you compare the squares on your dipstick with those on a colour chart. For example, consider the glucose square: this will darken according to the amount of glucose in the urine. Comparing the square to the colour chart the result will either be: no glucose, glucose trace, glucose +, glucose ++ or glucose +++. Make a note of the results of the test.

When should you test urine for glucose and ketones?

It can be helpful to use urine glucose monitoring regularly, as it may show that during a certain period of the day or night you start to excrete glucose. You can then do a blood glucose test to see what is happening. Also, it may be useful to use urine glucose monitoring in

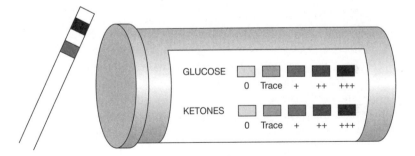

Figure 3 Urine testing – the dipstick illustrated reads glucose +++, ketones +

between blood monitoring, to see what is happening to your blood sugar level. Urine monitoring is also useful in a situation where you can't or don't want to use blood glucose monitoring.

You should monitor for urinary ketones:

- whenever your child feels unwell; ketones can make you feel hungry, nauseous or even make you sick;
- if the blood sugar level has been above about 15 mmol/l for more than two or three hours;
- whenever unwell with another illness such as a cold or diarrhoea; here the body may need more insulin than normal so your blood glucose levels might be higher than normal;
- in vomiting, one of the symptoms of high levels of ketones; vomiting, especially if without diarrhoea, is often due to a lack of insulin, resulting in high blood glucose levels which need treating.

In all these situations, the blood glucose level may be higher than normal. Checking the urinary ketones can show if the level is getting dangerously high.

What do the results mean?

Many people can become confused when looking at the results of the urine tests. The more + signs that your test shows, the more glucose or ketones there are in the blood.

Urine glucose and ketones

- No glucose or ketones (glucose 0, ketones 0) – normal results, though blood sugars might be low.
- Glucose but no ketones (glucose +, ++ or +++, and ketones 0) – probably high blood sugar level from too much glucose or too little insulin, but the body has not yet entered starvation mode, so levels are not dangerously high, but may become so.
- Glucose and ketones (glucose +, ++ or +++ *AND* ketones +, ++ or +++) – not enough insulin, levels of glucose might be getting dangerously high and need treating urgently with insulin to turn off the production of ketones.
- Ketones but no glucose (glucose 0, ketones +, ++ or +++) – the body may be producing starvation ketones from not having enough food.

If you test urine in the morning, on first waking, you cannot tell when any glucose or ketones were excreted. If your child has ketones but no glucose in the urine, she may need to eat more before going to bed. If your child wakes up with both glucose and ketones and is feeling sick, the likelihood is that she is currently producing ketones and so needs insulin treatment.

Is the reading correct?

The test may not work if the strips are out of date or the lid of the jar has been open too long so the strips have reacted with something in the atmosphere, so always check that the strips are in date. Certain drugs such as aspirin (which should not be given to children) may make the reading inaccurate.

Blood ketones

Some machines test for blood ketones. These are more accurate than urine ketone tests. Once insulin is given, the body stops producing ketones. You can see this quickly with a blood ketone test. However, ketones may still be found in the urine for some time after the body has stopped producing them, so the test is less accurate. The same rules apply as for urinary glucose and ketones.

> #### Blood glucose and ketones
> - High blood glucose and high blood ketones – these are diabetes ketones, you need more insulin.
> - High blood ketones and low blood glucose – these are starvation ketones, you need more food.

The HbA1c blood test

The finger-prick blood test described above shows your blood glucose currently, and the urine tests show the glucose over the last few hours. The HbA1c test shows the average blood glucose control over the last two to three months. HbA1c stands for glycosylated haemoglobin.

The red blood cells in the body contain haemoglobin that carries oxygen from the lungs to the rest of the cells in the body and then carries the carbon dioxide produced by these cells back to the lungs to be breathed out. Red blood cells are produced in the bone marrow and live for on average 120 days before they are destroyed by the spleen. Glucose can bind to the haemoglobin in the red blood cells. The amount of glucose that binds to the haemoglobin depends on the amount of glucose in the blood.

The HbA1c or glycosylated haemoglobin test measures how much of the haemoglobin in the red cells has glucose attached to it. It is expressed as a percentage; for example if the result is 10 per cent it means that 10 per cent of the haemoglobin has glucose bound to it and the other 90 per cent of the haemoglobin does not.

As the red cells live for about 120 days, the HbA1c test reflects the average blood glucose control over the last two to three months. It is important to note that it shows *average* blood glucose control. This means that your HbA1c test can have the same value if your blood glucose was at a constant level, or if you had many high and low readings, as they average out at the same level. This is why you cannot simply rely on a glycosylated haemoglobin test every three months but should also monitor your blood glucose daily. The test does not include the average readings in the week just before the test as at this time the bonds between the haemoglobin and glucose are not yet stable.

Fructosamine test

The fructosamine test is similar to the HbA1c test, in that it measures an average blood glucose over a period of time, in this case the preceding two to three weeks. Again a blood test is used to measure the glucose that has bound to proteins in the blood. As with the HbA1c test, if blood glucose levels are high, more binds to the proteins, and so the fructosamine test will have a higher value.

This test is used when the HbA1c test is unreliable, such as if a person has anaemia or when blood glucose levels are changing rapidly, like after starting a new treatment. It is not routinely used to monitor long-term glucose levels as it only represents an average of the previous two to three weeks and not the two to three months that can be seen with the HbA1c test.

Routine check-ups

Initially after diagnosis, you will see your doctors and diabetes team very regularly. Once things settle down, routine appointments tend to take place about every three months. It is at this appointment that the HbA1c test is taken and you have an opportunity to talk and ask questions about you or your child's diabetes and its control. At each appointment your child is weighed and measured to make sure that she is growing properly. Once a year, more detailed tests may be taken to check for other conditions, such as the level of fats, or other hormones in your blood. She will also have regular eye checks (see Chapter 8, 'Long-term complications').

Check-ups are an opportunity for you to work with your team to ensure that you have the best treatment possible for your diabetes.

Common questions

- *How is the test taken?* The HbA1c test is a blood test. It is not a finger-prick test; a sample of blood from a vein is needed, generally taken from the inside of the elbow or the band of the hand. Blood tests can be difficult, especially with younger children. Local anaesthetic creams or sprays can be used to numb the skin so the test is less painful.

   Blood tests can be distressing for the child who is having the test, but also for you, as the parent watching your child have something done that they don't like! Very young children have to be held very tightly during a blood test so that they don't struggle so the test can be carried out as quickly as possible. Some children do not like being held tightly and so cry as soon as they are held and sometimes not when the test is taken!

- *How often is the test taken?* A HbA1c test should be done every three months.

- *What should the HbA1c value be?* The percentage of HbA1c should be less than approximately 7 per cent. The exact range of values depends on the particular range your local hospital uses; these may vary slightly around the country. Studies have shown that values of less than 8 per cent reduce the risk of the complications of diabetes in the long term.

   During puberty, you may notice that your HbA1c rises by about 1 per cent. This rise can occur even if diabetes is controlled very well. During puberty the body secretes more growth hormone as it is a time of growth. As mentioned in Chapter 1 on the control of blood glucose, growth hormone acts to raise blood glucose.

- *What if the level is above 7–8 per cent?* This means that blood glucose has been on average higher than recommended over the preceding three months and therefore the risk of long-term complications is increased. Here, your team will advise you on any lifestyle or treatment changes that may be needed.

- *What if the level is below 6?* This means that blood glucose over the preceding three months has been on average lower than the recommended values. In this situation, hypoglycaemia may develop (see Chapter 7). Avoiding hypoglycaemia is important – the pay-off may be accepting slightly higher blood glucose levels to prevent hypoglycaemia occurring. Again, your team will advise you.

4

Insulin injections

For insulin to work, it needs to be in the bloodstream. Currently, the only way that you can give insulin is by injection. The thought of giving injections can be daunting, but they will soon be part of your daily routine. Perhaps the most important thing is to try and not be scared as your child picks up on this fear. Be as matter of fact as you can. You are not trying to hurt her, but to help by giving her the insulin that she needs. Your diabetes team will help you learn to give the injections.

It is normal for children to be apprehensive or scared of injections. Try letting them give their teddies or dolls injections; if you feel brave, give yourself an injection (*do not use insulin on yourself*, use sterile saline). Children can become involved in giving themselves insulin and blood monitoring from an early age. You can start by involving them in getting the equipment together such as by getting the insulin out of the fridge, to letting them hold the syringe or pen injector with you. By about eight or nine years old, most children can give themselves their insulin injections.

Where should you give insulin injections?

This question can be divided into three parts: which part of the body do you choose, how deep should the injection be given and where will cause the least pain? The insulin is injected into the skin, not directly into a vein, and once injected diffuses into the bloodstream.

Where on the body should you inject?

There are three main areas: the tummy or abdomen, the thigh or the buttocks. For injection purposes the tummy is the area around and below the belly button, the thigh the area of the leg between the knee and the groin crease, and the buttocks the upper outer area of the buttock (if you imagine each buttock has a clock face on it, the area between 12 and 3 o'clock on the right buttock, and between 9 and 12 o'clock on the left buttock).

Insulin injected into these areas is absorbed at different rates into the bloodstream. Insulin injected into the tummy is absorbed quicker and therefore works faster than insulin injected into the thigh. So a short-acting insulin should be injected into the tummy and a long- or intermediate-acting insulin should be injected into the thigh or buttocks. Very small children may not have a lot of tummy area so the buttocks may have to be used for short-acting insulin.

Always use the same area for the same type of insulin, so that you can get a predictable response in the blood sugars. Within each area you should move around a bit each day to avoid the side effect of getting lumps of fat under the skin (see side effects, below). Massaging the area after an injection increases the blood flow and so the insulin is absorbed quicker.

Remember:

- fast-acting insulin – inject into the tummy;
- intermediate- or long-acting insulin – inject into the thighs.

How deep should you inject?

The skin has many layers. The layer of fat immediately underneath the skin is called the subcutaneous region. Underneath the subcutaneous layer is muscle. You are aiming to inject into the subcutaneous layer and not into the muscle layer. This is because insulin is absorbed quicker from the muscle than from the subcutaneous region. Although this means that it works quicker, it also means that the effects of the insulin do not last very long. The doses and types of insulin used are worked out to allow for the slower absorption from the subcutaneous layer.

In order to inject into the subcutaneous layer, you should pinch a small area of skin between two fingers, to lift it up away from the muscle and then insert the needle into this flap of skin at about an angle of 45 degrees (see Figure 4). This method can be used with any needle.

How do you inject to cause the least pain?

First look at the end of a needle (called the bevil). It is not one point but has one very sharp end and a flatter edge (see Figure 4). You want to use the sharp pointed end to inject with as this causes less pain than the flatter edge. Turn the needle so the sharper edge is what enters the skin first. Also, inserting the needle quickly in one motion hurts less than slowly pushing it into the skin.

Some areas of the skin are more sensitive to touch and pain than others. This is due to the distribution of nerves in the skin; for example,

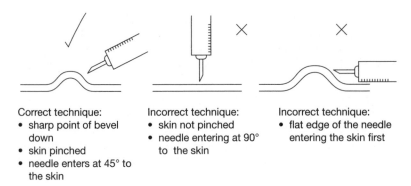

Correct technique:
- sharp point of bevel down
- skin pinched
- needle enters at 45° to the skin

Incorrect technique:
- skin not pinched
- needle entering at 90° to the skin

Incorrect technique:
- flat edge of the needle entering the skin first

Figure 4 Injection technique

the skin on your hands is much more sensitive than the skin on your arms or back as you need to have more sensation in your hands so that you can use them properly. Even within a certain area of the body, some places are more sensitive than others. You can try to test the areas that are more sensitive by touching your thigh or stomach all over with a needle; the places that are less sensitive may hurt less so you could try and use them for injections. Remember, you have to inject in a slightly different place each day to prevent side effects in the skin.

Different methods of injection

Depending on the type of insulin you use, you will need needles and syringes, or pen injectors, the different kinds of insulin themselves and somewhere to dispose of the needles. Everything you need will be supplied on prescription. You will not have to pay the prescription charge. Children under 16 do not pay prescription charges, and after that you will be given a payment exclusion card as people with diabetes do not pay for their prescriptions.

Needles and syringes

The traditional way of giving an injection is to draw up the solution into a syringe and then attach a needle to the syringe. The needle is inserted into the skin and the plunger of the syringe pushed down to inject the solution. Needles and syringes are still used to give insulin. Special syringes can be used that are marked with insulin units so you can measure the correct volume of insulin. Always wash your hands before drawing up or giving any injection.

Any long- or intermediate-acting insulin needs to be mixed before injecting otherwise crystals form in the insulin. Don't shake the bottle as it will cause air bubbles which are difficult to get rid of in the syringe. Mix the insulin by rolling the bottle about 20 times. Crystals can form in the solution and can block the needle, so try not to inject very slowly to prevent this occurring.

The dose of insulin is described in units (U) or international units (IU). The more units of insulin you give, the larger the dose. Most insulin is diluted to 100 units per millilitre of fluid; this is called the concentration of insulin. You should always check the concentration of the insulin in your bottles. How much fluid you draw up into the syringe will decide how many units will be given.

To draw up insulin into the syringe, follow the steps listed here.

- Check that the insulin has not passed its use by (expiry) date.
- Put a needle on the syringe and pull back on the plunger so air is drawn up into the syringe, up to the volume of insulin that you need.
- Leave that needle on the syringe and insert it through the top of the insulin bottle and then inject the air you have drawn up into the bottle.
- Turn the bottle upside down and pull back on the plunger of the syringe to draw up the amount of insulin you need.

If you need to inject a mixture of short- and long-acting insulin you need to draw them both up in the same syringe, using two different needles.

- Inject the relevant amount of air into the long-acting insulin bottle, then take the empty syringe away but leave the needle in the bottle.
- Using a second needle inject air into the short-acting bottle and then draw up the amount of short-acting insulin needed into the syringe.
- Then take the syringe (with some insulin in) and needle out of the short-acting insulin bottle and discard the needle.
- Attach the syringe to the needle that is left in the long-acting bottle. You don't need to inject air into it as you have already done it.
- Draw up the amount of long-acting insulin needed into the syringe.
- The two kinds of insulin can then be mixed in the syringe by rolling the syringe between your hands.
- Always draw up the short-acting insulin first, as if errors are made, it is safer this way.

To inject:

- Place a new clean needle on the syringe.
- Hold the syringe with the new needle facing upwards and tap it a few times to push out any air bubbles.
- The risk of skin infection is very small and so many people don't use an alcohol wipe to disinfect the skin before an injection as it increases the stinging sensation.
- Then, as described above, pinch a piece of skin on the tummy or thigh depending on what insulin is being used, and insert the needle at a 45-degree angle, sharpest edge first (see Figure 4), and push on the plunger to inject the insulin.
- Remove the needle and dispose of the needle and syringe safely.

Pen injections

Insulin pens are pre-loaded with enough insulin for repeated doses. There are various different types of pen injectors but all have a cartridge filled on average with about 300 units of a certain type of insulin and a needle for injection. You can adjust the dose of insulin given by turning a dial or clicking a button. They are very accurate, more accurate than drawing up the insulin by syringe. Unfortunately they are not available for all types of insulin. Pen injectors come in disposable, one-off doses and also in reusable forms (though you may have to replace the needle). If you use different pens for different types of insulin, for example pre-meal insulin and night-time insulin, you need to make sure that they look very different so you do not get confused between them and accidentally use the wrong pen.

- Check that the pen (and therefore the insulin it contains) has not passed its expiry date.
- If the pen contains a long-acting or intermediate-acting insulin, roll the pen between your hands about twenty times to mix the insulin.
- Set the dose to 1 to 2 units, hold the pen and needle upright and away from the body, and eject the insulin into the air by pressing the button. This is the test dose and ensures that the needle is full of insulin and not air and that the insulin is flowing correctly.
- Then set to the dose needed and as described above, pinch the skin between two fingers, insert the needle into the skin at a 45-degree angle and press the button to release the correct amount of insulin.
- Hold the needle in the skin for about 10 to 15 seconds to ensure all the insulin is given, otherwise sometimes a drop of insulin, perhaps

as much as a unit or two, may leak out of the needle after it has been taken out of the skin. This does not occur using syringes as you inject the entire contents of the syringe, while with a pen injector there is still insulin left for next time.

Unless you are using a single-dose disposable pen injector there will be insulin left in the pen for the next dose. You should replace the needle to prevent infections and also because the more times a needle is used, the blunter and therefore more painful it becomes. After each injection, replace the needle and before each injection do a test shot into the air to fill the needle with insulin and make sure there are no blockages.

Automatic injectors

An automatic injector is a machine that you press against the skin; on pressing a button the needle automatically pops out, enters the skin and an insulin dose is delivered. Some people find this easier than having to inject the needle themselves. Another form of automatic injector uses a jet: a thin jet of insulin is put under the skin using very high pressures. It does not use needles, which may be good if you are scared of needles, but it may not make a difference to whether or not the injection causes pain.

Indwelling catheters

An indwelling catheter is a very small piece of tubing that is inserted under the skin, generally into the tummy, and stays there for a few days. One side of the tube stays on the outside of the body and the other underneath the skin. Insulin can be injected through the tube so that a new injection does not need to be given every time. The end of the tube outside the body is covered to prevent any bacteria entering the body through the tube. The catheter can stay in for about five days before it needs to be changed. Not all kinds of insulin can be given through the catheter, but it can be used for short-acting insulin and for some of the longer-acting insulins.

Instead of giving an injection each time insulin is needed, the insulin is drawn up or a pen used as described above, the plastic covering the open end of the catheter is cleaned and then the insulin injected into the tube with a needle. This is not painful as it does not involve injecting the skin. If this method is used, you will be taught how to insert new indwelling catheters. Inserting an indwelling catheter may be more painful than a simple insulin injection so a local anaesthetic cream is used. The skin must be cleaned to decrease the risk of infection.

Indwelling catheters can be good in young children and in the early stages after diagnosis to help them to get used to treatment without regular (painful) injections. However, possible problems with indwelling catheters include itching from the plaster around the catheter and scars from having lots of catheters in the skin over time. There is also an increased risk of infection in the skin around the catheter site as there is a continuous connection between the outside world (with all its bacteria and viruses) and the inside of the body. Older children may not want to look different from their peers and so may not like to have a catheter which can be seen on the outside of the body.

Insulin pumps

An insulin pump is a device that is continually attached to the body via a small needle and gives a continuous dose of insulin. It is also called a continuous subcutaneous insulin infusion. It consists of a small needle placed under the skin, which is attached via a small plastic tube to the pump. The pump itself is small and contains enough insulin for at least 24 hours, before it will need refilling. Most pumps deliver a continuous basal rate and can deliver extra pre-meal boluses as needed. Insulin pumps deliver insulin to the body in a way that most closely mimics the natural secretion of insulin from the pancreas. As such, if used correctly, it should give the best control of blood glucose.

The needle is inserted into the abdomen (or, less commonly, the buttocks) and the small pump is then carried, strapped to the body, attached to a belt, or carried in a bag. Every few days, the needle and infusion set need to be changed, and the insertion site should be rotated. The pump is generally worn 24 hours a day, through the night. The pump itself can be removed for contact sports or showering or swimming (though some pumps are now waterproof), but the needle and tubing are left in place. Pumps can only be disconnected for a short period of time, up to one hour. You still need to carry extra insulin, either in pen injectors or with needles and syringes in case the pump stops working.

Pumps are more expensive than treatment with pen injections or needles and syringes. As such, there are criteria within the NHS as to the situations where a pump should be offered. These criteria have been decided by NICE (National Institute for Health and Clinical Excellence). As with all NICE guidelines, the criteria will be reviewed in the future and may change. Currently in the UK, insulin pumps are an option for treatment for people with type 1 diabetes if multiple injection regimens have not given good control of blood glucose levels without regular serious hypoglycaemic episodes *and* if the patient is able and willing to use the pump properly and successfully. If you do not meet these criteria but feel that an insulin pump would be the best form of treatment to improve your quality of life, then it is possible to buy a pump privately. At the time of writing this costs about £2,000 for the pump, and then about £1,000 per year for the non-reusable parts such as needles and infusion sets.

The advantages of using a pump are related to the good diabetic control it gives, hopefully preventing hypoglycaemia or hyperglycaemia. A pump also gives you more flexibility regarding meals and exercise. The disadvantages of using a pump include the fact that they use short-acting insulin. These means that you will not have a store of insulin within the body and if the supply from the pump is cut off for whatever reason, you are at risk of developing insulin deficiency, hyperglycaemia and ketoacidosis relatively quickly. Therefore, you can only be disconnected from the pump for about up to one hour and have to do very regular blood glucose monitoring throughout the day. The pump is carried or strapped to the body and cannot always be hidden, for example during changing. You may find that your child does not want to look different to his or her peers and so would find a pump difficult.

Finally the pump acts as a continuous reminder that you have diabetes and need treatment. For some people, this is an advantage, it reminds them to eat correctly and look after themselves; for others, this continuous reminder is a disadvantage.

Discarding needles

The used needles from the syringes or pens need to be disposed of safely. You should not simply put them in a bin bag as the needles are sharp and can poke out through the bag and could hurt someone. You will be given a 'sharps box', a special box for used needles and syringes that can then be safely disposed of.

How do you store insulin?

Insulin can be stored at room temperature (about 20 degrees Celsius). Any insulin not used after a month of being stored at room temperature should be discarded as it begins to lose strength. Insulin should not be exposed to extreme heat or cold as it begins to lose strength if stored at temperatures below 2 degrees and above 25 degrees Celsius. Insulin can be kept in normal daylight but not in direct sunlight, so put it in a shaded place in the car or wrap it in something wet.

You should keep spare insulin in the fridge, but could keep the current bottle or pen you are using out of the fridge if you preferred, as it would be used shortly. Don't put spare insulin in the fridge too near the freezer as it needs to be above 2 degrees Celsius. Discard any insulin that has been kept out of the fridge for over a month or has passed its use-by date.

What are the potential side effects of insulin injections?

In all areas of medicine, the potential benefits of any treatment must be weighed up against any potential side effects. In diabetes, potential side effects are balanced against no treatment, which would result in high blood glucose levels, increasing the risk of long-term, potentially life-threatening, complications.

The side effects of insulin treatment can be divided into those relating to the injection itself and those relating to the insulin.

Side effects of injecting into the skin

- *Pain* See above for how to minimize the pain of injections.
- *Bruises* Bruises are due to small amounts of bleeding under the skin. They disappear as the body absorbs the blood. As you inject the insulin the needle may go through a tiny blood vessel that may then bleed and cause a bruise. These blood vessels are very small and the body automatically limits any bleeding. The bruise should go away in a few days.

Side effects related to insulin

- *Hypoglycaemia* If too much insulin is injected it can lead to hypoglycaemia. Low blood glucose levels make you feel unwell and can be dangerous at very low levels. See Chapter 7, 'Diabetic emergencies'.
- *Skin irritation* The skin can become red and itchy after an injection. You may have a reaction or allergy to the metal of the needle, a preservative used in the insulin or the insulin itself. Tests can be carried out to confirm whether or not you have an allergy. The symptoms tend to improve with time as the body gets used to the injections. If the reaction is severe, your doctor may prescribe antihistamine tablets to help.
- *Lumps and bumps in the skin* Insulin encourages fatty tissue to grow. Regular injections of insulin may lead to fatty lumps growing under the skin, called lipohypertrophy. They can be prevented by slightly

changing the site of your injections regularly. Injecting into these lumps may be less painful but the insulin is absorbed more slowly and this has an effect on your blood glucose levels. Sometimes the opposite occurs, called lipoatrophy, where a shallow space like a crater appears under the skin. Why they occur is not yet known.

- *Insulin antibodies* Antibodies are part of the body's defence system against infection. They are produced whenever the body meets a substance that it does not recognize as its own, for example if it meets the cold virus. Insulin may be recognized as 'foreign', and insulin antibodies may form so that the insulin cannot work. Antibodies used to be a much bigger problem when insulin from cows or pigs was used to treat diabetes. Nowadays human insulin is used (insulin with exactly the same chemical structure as that found in humans) and so it is relatively rare to have a significant problem with insulin antibodies.

5

Treatment of diabetes

Type 1 diabetes

In type 1 diabetes, the pancreas does not produce insulin. In someone without diabetes, there is a constant secretion of a small amount of insulin, throughout the day and night: the 'basal' insulin. When a meal or snack is eaten, the levels of glucose within the blood rise and so more insulin is produced to cope with this, called the insulin 'boluses'. As the blood glucose levels fall, the secretion of insulin returns to the lower basal levels.

The aim of treatment is to replace the body's natural production of insulin with insulin injections. There are various different regimes, using different types of insulin. The aim is to mimic the natural production of insulin as closely as possible. The body normally works very well to keep the blood glucose within a very small range. A good treatment regimen aims to do the same, but without putting the person at too high a risk of hypoglycaemic attacks.

Types of insulin

Generally human insulin is used in the treatment of diabetes – not insulin produced and donated by someone else, but insulin which is synthetic, produced in a laboratory, and has exactly the same chemical structure as the insulin naturally produced in the human body. This means that the body is more likely to recognize the insulin and less likely to reject it as 'foreign' and create antibodies against it.

Synthetic insulin is divided into different types depending on how fast- or slow-acting it is. The insulin produced naturally by the pancreas is not divided into fast- and slow-acting – the body regulates the speed and length of response to the insulin by how much it secretes. However, to reproduce that in diabetes would require many, many injections throughout the day, so insulins with different speeds and length of action are used.

- *Short-acting or soluble insulin* – for example, actrapid insulin – is insulin without anything added to make it last longer. It is the same as that produced by the pancreas. It is given to mimic the bolus secretions of insulin in the body. It is given before mealtimes as it takes 20 to 30 minutes to start working. Its effects last only about five hours. This insulin is a clear solution (if it has turned cloudy it should not be used).

- *Rapid-acting insulin* – for example, NovoRapid insulin. This works even faster than normal short-acting insulin as it has already been broken down into its active parts. It starts working almost straight away and generally within about ten minutes. It lasts about one hour. It can also be used in between mealtimes to act on high blood glucose levels.

- *Long-acting insulin* – for example, glargine insulin. Additives are mixed with the insulin so it is released slowly and the effects are long lasting but not as intense. The additives make the insulin cloudy and need mixing by rolling between your hands before injecting. If the insulin has lumps in it, it should not be used. Depending on the type of long-acting insulin, they can work up to over a 24-hour period, giving a slow and steady effect.

- *Intermediate-acting insulin* – for example, insulatard insulin – has some additives delaying its effect but not as many as in long-acting insulins. It has properties in between those of short-acting and long-acting insulins. It can be used to mimic the basal secretion of insulin, but two injections per day may need to be given. Intermediate-acting insulin is also cloudy and needs mixing before use. If there are lumps in the liquid, discard that bottle.

- *Intravenous insulin* – short-acting insulin is injected directly into a vein and the bloodstream, instead of subcutaneously, and so works very quickly. It is also used up very quickly, in about three or four minutes, and so continuous infusion of insulin into the vein is needed; a 'drip' of insulin is used. Intravenous insulin is not used for home treatment. It is generally used in the treatment of diabetic ketoacidosis in hospital, or during an operation, where very exact control of blood glucose is needed.

A combination of short- and longer-acting insulins is generally used to try and copy the natural insulin secretion by the pancreas, reflecting the basal and peaks of secretion as closely as possible. Apart from with rapid-acting insulins, the bigger the dose of insulin you use, the stronger and longer lasting its effects will be.

Different insulin regimes

The different insulin regimes described below use different mixtures of shorter- and longer-acting insulins throughout the day to keep blood glucose levels in the correct range. The regimen that is best for your

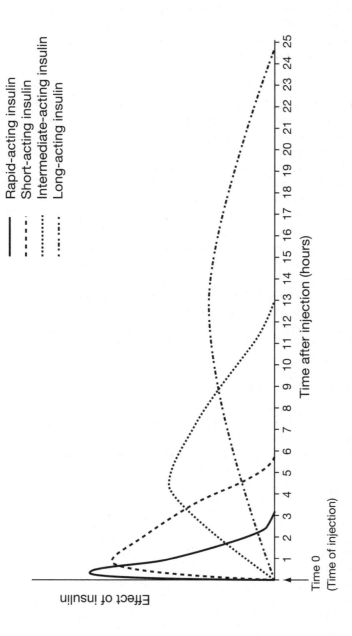

Figure 5 The timescale of action of different insulins

Rapid-acting insulin
Short-acting insulin
Intermediate-acting insulin
Long-acting insulin

Effect of insulin

Time 0
(Time of injection)

Time after injection (hours)

child depends on how much insulin she needs in the day, what she eats and the physical activity that she does, as well as how many injections you are prepared to give, all weighed up against the need for the best blood glucose control possible. You can change treatment regimes, but this should not be done without the advice of your diabetic team.

Two injections per day

Also known as twice-daily treatment, this is a common form of treatment. Two injections are given per day, one in the morning before breakfast and the other before the evening meal. The total amount of insulin needed in a day is calculated; two-thirds of this total amount is given in the morning and the remaining one-third given at the evening meal. Let's assume your child's daily requirement of insulin is 24 units: in this twice-daily regime, 16 units is given in the morning and 8 units at night. Mixtures of short- and intermediate-acting insulins are generally used to last throughout the day.

If the total amount of insulin needed throughout the day is very large, then large doses are needed, increasing the risk of hypoglycaemia, and so more snacks may be needed. Also, if the dose of insulin at night is not enough, your child may become hyperglycaemic during the night or in the morning. Twice-daily treatment is simple to remember and easy to carry out. However, you do not have very much control, as once the insulin has been given it acts on the body, no matter what your child has eaten or how much physical activity he has done that day.

Three injections per day

Also known as thrice-daily or three-dose treatment. As with twice-daily treatment, two-thirds of the total daily insulin dose is given in the morning and a mixture of short and intermediate acting insulins are used. However, the evening mealtime dose is divided, before the meal only the short-acting insulin is given to tide you over after the effects of eating a meal. You then give the third injection of the day at night, just before going to bed. This third injection is of an intermediate-acting insulin, which should then act throughout the night.

This regime is useful if you find that your child is regularly getting morning hyperglycaemia on a twice-daily treatment regime. In that case, he was not having enough insulin throughout the night, but, increasing the dose of the second injection would increase the risk of hypoglycaemia. Splitting the second dose into two separate injections, as described in the three-injections-daily treatment aims to prevent this. However, as with a two-injections-daily regime, once the insulin is given, you have very little control over its effect.

Four or more injections per day – basal bolus regime

Giving multiple (four or more) injections per day gives the most amount of control of your blood glucose levels. However, the good control has to be weighed up against having to give more injections.

In this regimen, injections are given before each main meal and also before bed. The pre-meal injections are of a short-acting insulin to act as the boluses of insulin. If you have a night-time snack, another injection of a short-acting insulin is needed. A long-acting insulin is then given at night, or an intermediate insulin both at night and in the morning to mimic the basal secretion of insulin. This regimen is called a 'basal bolus' regime.

This regime allows you to adjust how much insulin before each meal, depending on current blood sugar levels, what and how much you intend to eat, and the level of physical activity you do in the day.

If you are using a short-acting insulin as your pre-meal bolus injection, you need to give the insulin about 30 minutes before eating so it will be working when the meal is digested and the glucose enters the bloodstream. If you are using a rapid-acting insulin as your pre-meal bolus you can take the insulin just before eating as it only takes about 10 minutes to work. Once the short-acting insulin is given, your child must eat in the next half an hour to an hour as otherwise she is at risk of developing hypoglycaemia. You have more control over when you eat with a rapid-acting insulin as you inject just before you start your meal.

Pre-breakfast doses of insulin need to be higher than the other pre-meal injections, due to the effect of the increased secretion of growth hormone throughout the night (growth hormone acts to increase blood sugar levels – the dawn phenomenon), and because breakfast contains a higher proportion of carbohydrates, such as cereal, compared to other meals.

Among other factors, how much insulin is given, the combination of the different insulins used, what you eat and how much physical activity you do all affect blood glucose level. Monitoring blood glucose before and two hours after a meal helps you decide the dose of insulin needed or if a snack is needed.

How much insulin do I give?

Initially, your doctor and diabetic team will advise you how much insulin is needed over a 24-hour period and how the doses should be divided up. If your child has been unwell and required admission to hospital, she may have been on an insulin drip for at least 24 hours, even after she got better. The doctors can then calculate how many units of insulin were used and therefore how much insulin is needed. Often, a lot more insulin is needed at the beginning of treatment than later on. For regimes that involve two or three injections per day, you give two-thirds of the total day's insulin in the morning, for other regimes you give a proportion of the day's total dose before each meal and at night. You will be advised how much insulin to use.

The same amount of insulin will not give the same effects in different people, as different people are more or less sensitive to insulin. Generally, smaller children are more sensitive to insulin; they also weigh less and so less insulin is needed when compared to an older child. Other factors that affect sensitivity to insulin include stress and physical illness, exercise, weight gain or loss, puberty and recent blood glucose levels (see Figure 6). If your child has had a day of high blood glucose levels she will have become slightly resistant to insulin and so will need more insulin to bring the level back to the normal range; conversely low blood glucose levels increase the body's sensitivity to insulin. Do not worry that as your child gets older she needs more insulin: this is to be expected as she grows.

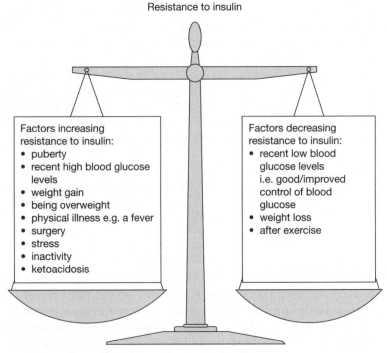

Figure 6 Factors affecting resistance to insulin

The amount of insulin needed in a day is continually changing depending on the factors mentioned above as well as what is eaten and the level of physical activity. There is no 'perfect' insulin dose; what is perfect is a changing dose dependent on your child's need.

Changing the insulin dose

Learning to take control over your insulin dosage is initially difficult, but your team will be able to advise you.

If you are using a twice- or three-times-daily regime and notice that your child is regularly getting afternoon hyperglycaemia, you may need to increase the morning dose. Alternatively, if morning hypoglycaemia is a problem, you may need to reduce the night-time dose.

The explanation below refers to a multiple injection or basal bolus regimen. You should test blood glucose before each meal (at least half an hour before mealtimes for short-acting insulins, ten minutes before mealtimes for rapid-acting insulins), to help you decide how much insulin to inject. You also need to weigh up what your child is going to eat against what she is going to do after the meal. If you know that she is going to eat a carbohydrate-rich meal such as pasta, or that she is hungry and will eat more than usual, it would be reasonable to give a slightly higher dose of insulin than usual. However, if you are serving pasta because the afternoon involves a lot of physical activity such as cycling or running around with friends, then the carbohydrate is used up by this activity and so the insulin dose should not be increased.

Alternatively, if your child is doing a lot of exercise but does not feel like eating more, you could consider decreasing her insulin dose, or having regular snacks to prevent hypoglycaemia. If you know she will be resting, this also should be taken into account, as resting does not use up as much glucose as exercise.

Carbohydrate counting is a method of calculating how much insulin is needed depending on what you are going to eat (see Chapter 6, 'Diet and staying well').

You need to take into account your child's current blood glucose reading. If she has a high blood glucose reading and is about to eat a meal, then more insulin may be needed. If she has a low blood glucose reading you may wish to decrease the insulin dose, or she could eat a bit more than originally planned. You should not attempt to decrease blood glucose level by not eating – food is needed for energy and growth, and not eating also puts your child at an increased risk of developing hypoglycaemia. The effect of changing your insulin dose depends on all the factors above, but also whether or not there is any intermediate- or long-acting insulin still within the body.

Finally, look back in your diary of blood glucose readings. Perhaps you have been in a similar situation before – what did you do then and how did it affect the blood glucose reading? Did changing the dose lead to hypoglycaemia? In this way, you can learn from previous episodes so that you make the most appropriate decision.

You should aim for blood glucose readings between 4 and 10 mmol/l. As glucose occurs naturally within the body, it is a balancing act – on one side of the scales are things acting to bring the blood glucose up to high levels such as food, on the other side of the scales are things acting to bring the blood glucose levels down, such as insulin and physical exercise (see Figure 7).

It is not advisable to increase an insulin dose by more than 0.1 unit/kg at a time at home. This means that if your child weighs 30 kg, you should not increase the insulin by more than 3 units as it would increase the risk of hypoglycaemia. In reality, changes to the dose are often even smaller. If your child's normal dose is less than 3 units, changes of half a unit can be made; if her dose is normally between

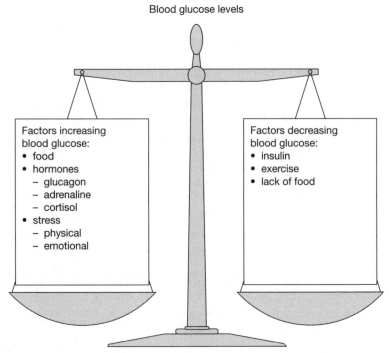

Figure 7 The balancing act of blood glucose control

3 and 10 units, you could consider changing by up to 1 unit; if her normal dose is more than 10 units, you could change by up to 2 units. It is better to adjust insulin doses slowly, over a period of time, to decrease the risk of hypoglycaemia.

You should not change the dose of insulin with every blood glucose reading. It is normal to have some variation in blood glucose reading, especially if your child is not drinking enough water as the blood becomes more concentrated. Unless you know that you have a specific change in mind, such as a lot of physical exercise, illness, a special meal or event that involves eating a lot such as a birthday party, don't change the doses too regularly. Wait a few days, and if blood sugar levels are consistently high two hours after lunchtime for a few days, then it is reasonable to slightly increase the insulin dose.

If you consistently find that your child's blood glucose readings are high before she goes to bed, you could try increasing or giving an extra dose of a rapid-acting insulin. Consistently high blood glucose levels in the morning can be due to the dawn phenomenon of increased growth hormone secretion during the night increasing blood glucose levels, a rebound phenomenon from hypoglycaemia during the night (also called the Somogyi phenomenon) or not enough insulin. Hyperglycaemia in the morning can be difficult to manage, so you should discuss this with your diabetes team.

You will quickly become used to changing the dose of the pre-meal short- or rapid-acting insulin. However, changing the dose of the intermediate- or longer-acting insulin is harder as you do not see the effects in the following few hours. Changing an intermediate-acting insulin has an effect that lasts many hours, up to a 24-hour period with long-acting insulins. It may be sensible to ask for advice from your diabetic team before changing the dosage of your basal (intermediate- or long-acting) insulin.

Finally, don't change everything at once. If you change both the dose of your night-time intermediate- or long-acting insulin, as well as changing the dose of your rapid- or short-acting insulin before each meal, it will rapidly become confusing. It will not be possible to determine which change in insulin dose is resulting in the change in blood glucose. Change one thing a small amount at a time, over a period of days. Changing blood glucose levels slowly is better, even if it means that you have high blood sugar levels for a few days, than risking severe hypoglycaemia. Remember, when changing doses, check blood glucose levels before and two hours after each meal, or whenever your child feels unwell.

Honeymoon phase

The honeymoon or remission phase of diabetes commonly occurs soon after diabetes has been diagnosed. Before diagnosis, your child will have had high levels of blood glucose for a while, which makes the body less sensitive to insulin. When diabetes is first diagnosed, high levels of insulin are often needed to overcome the body's resistance to the insulin. However, soon the body becomes sensitive to insulin again, and initially the pancreas may start to secrete some insulin again, so the amount of insulin needed from injections falls.

If you need less than 0.5 units/kg of your body weight per day (so if you weigh 35 kg and need less than 17.5 units of insulin a day) you have entered the honeymoon phase. As the pancreas is producing some insulin you may need to decrease the insulin doses, or even leave out the lunchtime or dinnertime doses. Hypoglycaemia is less likely during the remission phase as the pancreas tries to act as normal to regulate blood glucose. This means that if you inject some insulin and blood sugars fall, the pancreas decreases the insulin production to prevent hypoglycaemia.

Not everyone has a honeymoon phase. It does not mean that your child no longer has diabetes, as the honeymoon tends to last only about six months. A couple of years after diagnosis, the majority of people stop producing any insulin of their own and get all their insulin from injections. Once the honeymoon phase is over, insulin requirements rise.

Puberty

During puberty children grow very quickly and need more insulin. High levels of growth hormone are produced in the body to trigger this growth. Growth hormone is one of the hormones that also increase blood glucose levels. Levels of insulin produced by those without diabetes are increased during this time to balance the effects of the growth hormone. In diabetes, insulin doses need to be increased to counteract this spurt in growth hormone, even if diet and exercise habits have not changed.

The amount of insulin needed changes throughout puberty, according to when 'growth spurts' take place – this is when the most insulin is needed, as the most growth hormone is being produced.

Good control of diabetes is also important at this time to ensure that children meet their 'growth potential', that is, that they are as tall as they were expected to be. Routine check-ups include measuring height and weight to check growth. With good diabetic control, growth should be normal.

After puberty, insulin requirements stabilize at adult levels and fluctuate according to diet, activities and lifestyle.

Common questions regarding insulin treatment
When should you give the mealtime insulin?

This depends on whether short-acting or rapid-acting insulin is used. It does not matter if a mixture of intermediate-acting insulin is also injected at the same time as this takes some time to take effect. Different brands and types of insulin start working after differing periods of time but in general short-acting insulin should be injected 30 minutes before a meal, rapid-acting insulin 10 minutes before a meal (or occasionally even just before the meal). This time lag gives the insulin a chance to start working by the time the food is digested and blood glucose levels begin to rise.

I've given the insulin, but unavoidably the meal is delayed, what should I do?

It is important to plan meals and therefore times of insulin injections in advance; however, inevitably things happen, and a delayed mealtime may be unavoidable. In this situation you have insulin in the bloodstream but no food, and therefore no glucose to counteract it. Without food the risk of hypoglycaemia is significant: therefore give snacks or glucose energy drinks. Look for the symptoms of hypoglycaemia and act on them promptly (see Chapter 7, 'Diabetic emergencies').

When do you give the night-time insulin?

Again, this depends on the type of night-time insulin. The very long-acting insulins take a few hours to start working and so are taken with a mixture of a shorter-acting insulin before the evening meal. With intermediate-acting insulins it may be appropriate to take them before the evening snack or bedtime. Your team will advise you depending on the particular types and combination of insulins used.

I've given the insulin, but now my child won't finish her meal, what should I do?

Children often eat unpredictably. It can be difficult to know how much insulin to give before a meal. Do not wait until after a meal to decide how much insulin to give once you have seen how much your child has eaten, as it takes time for the insulin to start working (so she would have a period of hyperglycaemia after each meal).

If you have given a dose of insulin and your child eats less than expected, there is a risk of developing hypoglycaemia as the insulin still works but there is less glucose in the blood. Be aware of the symptoms of hypoglycaemia and act appropriately. To prevent this, you could offer a snack earlier than usual, or juice with the meal.

If your child regularly does not finish meals and eats slowly or eats a bit, stops for a few minutes and starts again, you could consider using a rapid-acting insulin and inject about halfway through the meal when you have an idea of how much your child is eating. This way, the rapid-acting insulin should work by the time the child finishes – hopefully within about ten minutes. A further option is to give your child a small dose of insulin corresponding to a small portion of food prior to the meal. If your child then eats more than normal, you can then give extra insulin as there is already some working in the blood from the first injection.

Teachers need to be aware of whether or not your child eats a full meal, so that snacks or cartons of juice can be offered if appropriate. Ask for a school menu and talk to your child about what she does and doesn't like, as if she doesn't like it, she won't eat it! Discuss with the school if there are options on the days that your child doesn't like the food available, or whether she could always be offered extra bread or juice. If she doesn't eat at mealtimes, she may be hungry later and need snacks.

If you are using a twice- or three-times-daily regime, you do not give a dose before each meal. Offer snacks or juices while waiting for the meal to compensate for the insulin already given.

Finally, if your child is not eating then she may be telling you that she has high blood sugars which can make her not feel hungry. Blood glucose levels should be checked before each meal with the finger-pricking device so that insulin doses can be adjusted accordingly. Alternatively she may not be hungry if she is unwell – see Chapter 6, 'Diet and staying well'.

Can you miss a meal?

If you have already given the pre-meal dose of insulin it is not advisable to miss a meal entirely as it increases the risk of hypoglycaemia – see the previous question. If a meal is missed, the body attempts to keep the blood glucose levels steady by producing glucose from the stores in the liver. So, even if you have not given the pre-meal dose of insulin and want to miss a meal, the body still needs some insulin, though less than if you had eaten.

If you are on a basal bolus regime you will have given your child a long- or intermediate-acting insulin to represent this basal secretion of insulin by the pancreas. Therefore, in this situation, as long as her blood glucose level is normal, if she is going to miss a meal, she should also miss the corresponding dose of rapid- or short-acting insulin. Note though, that she may become hypoglycaemic and need snacks later on. Alternatively, she may be very hungry and eat more at her next meal and need to adjust the next insulin dose accordingly.

If you use a treatment regime that involves injections of a short-acting insulin before meals you still need to give some insulin even if your child does not intend to eat. This is because short-acting insulin lasts for about five hours and acts as the basal secretion of insulin between meals. She needs less short-acting insulin than if she were going to eat, but some insulin should still be given.

If blood glucose level is high, do not let your child skip a meal in an attempt to lower the levels back to the normal range. If, however, levels are high and she wants to miss a meal for other reasons then she still needs a dose of insulin to lower the blood glucose. She could take less than normal, or eat snacks later to compensate. If her blood glucose level is low, it is not advisable to miss a meal; and if there is not time to eat a meal, she needs a snack or juice to prevent hypoglycaemia.

Missing meals increases the risk of hypoglycaemia, and your child should not miss more than one meal or snack in a row. Be aware of hypoglycaemia symptoms and see that your child eats if necessary (see Chapter 7, 'Diabetic emergencies').

Do you have to eat meals at the same time each day?

If you use a basal bolus regime, the long-acting insulin prevents insulin deficiency, giving you more flexibility about mealtimes. If not, then you need to be stricter, and your child needs to eat at approximately the same times each day, give or take an hour. If you are using regular short-acting insulin without a basal insulin it is necessary to eat every five hours as otherwise the effects of the short-acting insulin run out and blood glucose levels rise. If a meal is not eaten, consider snacks or juices.

My child does not want to eat proper meals, just a little bit every couple of hours. How do I manage this?

It depends what regime you are on. If you are using a twice- or three-times-daily regime, the mixture of short- and intermediate-acting insulin may need to be changed. Here it may be more appropriate to be on a basal bolus multiple-injection regimen as this gives more control over how much insulin is given prior to each 'mini meal'. Not all snacks or mini meals have the same effect on blood glucose readings.

Sugary snacks cause a sharp rise in blood glucose levels. Snacks containing more complex carbohydrates such as a granary bread sandwich, or those higher in protein or fat, lead to a slower rise in blood sugars. See Chapter 6, 'Diet and staying well'.

Why does giving the same dose of insulin not always have the same effect on blood glucose levels?

This does not mean that you are giving an inaccurate dose of insulin. The insulin has differing effects depending on many things ranging from the site of injection to a person's physical well-being. How and where the insulin is injected into the body affects how quickly it works – for example, it is absorbed more quickly via the tummy (see Chapter 4, 'Insulin injections'). Blood supply to the skin is increased by heat such as from a hot bath and decreased by cold, so on a hot day the insulin is absorbed more quickly. Exercise and massage increase the blood flow to the skin and also mean the insulin works faster. Injecting into the fatty lumps of lipohypertrophy (see side effects of insulin treatment on p. 37) or into areas that have a thick layer of fat under the skin slow down the absorption of insulin, so take longer to work. Other factors increase the body's resistance to insulin so it is less effective. These include stress, being physically unwell, such as having a temperature or having an operation, recent high blood glucose levels, puberty and weight gain. Factors that decrease the body's resistance to insulin, so that less insulin is needed, include exercise, losing weight and recent low blood glucose levels.

It is frustrating that you can get different results from the same amount of insulin, even if the same amount and type of food is eaten. In your diary, alongside where you note down daily blood glucose values, you could also document other things such as the site of injection, whether your child was unwell or particularly stressed, about to do exercise etc. This allows you to interpret previous blood glucose results more fully so you can use them to predict your child's response to a certain insulin dose in a certain situation.

What should you do if you forget a dose in a twice- or three-times-daily regimen?

In twice- or three-times-daily regimes you will probably use a mixture of short- and intermediate-acting insulins. If you use pre-mixed pen injectors you cannot adjust the mix, you can only adjust the total dose given. However, if you mix your own insulins with a needle and syringe, it is possible to use less or more of one kind of insulin. The aim in any situation where you miss an injection is to minimize the risk of hyperglycaemia due to insulin deficiency, which if very severe can become serious.

If you forget the morning dose of insulin and use a pre-mixed pen insulin, you could give a lower dose than normal. Alternatively, you could miss out the injection of pre-mixed insulin and just give regular doses of short-acting insulin until the next dose is due.

If you forget the morning dose and mix your own insulin you could adjust the mixture. If you remember immediately after eating, then reduce the dose of short-acting insulin by a small amount and keep the amount of intermediate-acting insulin at the normal dose as you need it to represent the basal insulin secretion until your next meal. If you remember a few hours after eating, you need to decrease the short-acting insulin much more, perhaps by half (as you are halfway to the next meal) and also decrease the dose of intermediate-acting insulin (perhaps by about a quarter), again as some time has elapsed so less is needed until the next dose. If you don't remember until your next meal, then use just short-acting insulin to tide you over until the next dose is due. Your team can advise how much the dose should be dropped as it will be a proportion of the total dose.

If you forget the evening dose but remember before going to bed, then give a smaller dose of intermediate-acting insulin. This is because there is less time until the next meal and next insulin injection and you do not want the effects of the night-time insulin dose to last longer than expected. You may need some short- or rapid-acting insulin with the evening snack in this situation. You could wake up during the night to check your child's blood glucose level.

What should you do if you forget to give the mealtime insulin in a basal bolus regime?

If you remember straight away you could give the insulin (especially if you use rapid-acting insulin). The more time that passes from when the injection was due, the less you should give. So, if you remember straight after the meal you might decrease the dose by only a small percentage, but if you remember a few hours after, you might decrease the dose by much more. If you miss an injection entirely, check the blood glucose level before your next meal as you may need to give a higher dose than usual before this meal.

What should you do if you forget the night-time insulin in a basal bolus regime?

If you wake up in the night and remember that you have not given your child her bedtime intermediate-acting insulin, you could give a smaller dose than normal. You can decrease the dose by about one or two units per hour. This means that if you normally give 16 units at 9 p.m. and wake up at 1 a.m. realizing you have forgotten the injection, you are four hours late, so should decrease the dose by 4 to 8 units.

If you wake and remember but it is less than five hours before you normally wake up and eat breakfast, you could leave out the night-time dose, measure your child's blood glucose and give her a small dose of short-acting insulin to tide her over until breakfast.

If you normally use a long-acting insulin at night, you can give it a few hours late, though you may need a small dose of short-acting insulin in the meantime. If you do not remember until the morning then half the dose should be taken to last until the next evening dose.

I have forgotten an injection and my child doesn't feel well, what should I do?

If your child does not feel well then you should check his blood glucose levels and also check his urine (or blood) for ketones. It may be that he has become so insulin deficient that he is developing ketoacidosis (see Chapter 7, 'Diabetic emergencies'). If he has both hyperglycaemia and ketones you need to give more insulin – in this situation, rapid-acting insulin should be used if possible. The maximum recommended dose to be given at home is 0.1 units per kilogram of body weight (i.e. in a weight of 45 kg, the maximum dose is 4.5 units of NovoRapid) to prevent severe hypoglycaemia. Test the blood glucose again after an hour; the dose can be repeated if your child's blood glucose level has not decreased two hours after the first injection.

You could contact your team for advice. If your child starts feeling nauseous, vomits, develops abdominal pain or other symptoms, if his blood glucose does not fall despite insulin, or you just feel that the situation is beyond your control, then go to your doctor or nearest hospital.

What should you do if you have given the wrong type of insulin by mistake?

To try and prevent this, ensure your insulin bottles or pens are clearly marked or look very different so you can easily tell them apart. Don't rely on the fact that most short-acting insulins are clear and long- or intermediate-acting insulins are cloudy as there are some newer long-acting insulins which are clear and short-acting insulin may go cloudy (in which case it should not be used).

If a long or intermediate acting insulin is taken during the day instead of the pre-meal short- or rapid-acting insulin, you will not see the effects straight away. It will not start working in time to have an effect on blood glucose related to that meal, so your child needs to take a small dose of his short-acting insulin as well (about half the dose is reasonable). Take the blood glucose regularly throughout the day, as you may need to decrease the amount of short-acting insulin taken before the next meal or give snacks to prevent hypoglycaemia.

If you give short-acting insulin at night when you should have given a longer-acting insulin, monitor for signs of hypoglycaemia and check blood glucose levels during the night. You probably need to give extra snacks to prevent hypoglycaemia. The effects of short-acting insulin wear off after about five hours so you will still need to give some inter-mediate- or long-acting insulin. Wait a few hours before giving the insulin and use a lower dose than normal.

Remember, mistakes happen, children eat more or less than expected, or sneak extra snacks, and we are all forgetful sometimes. It is not a disaster and you should not treat it as such. Simply watch for the symptoms and signs of hypoglycaemia or ketoacidosis, measure blood glucose levels regularly and act appropriately. Do not panic if one reading is higher or lower than expected, as a one-off high reading does not automatically hugely increase the risk of long-term complications. It is common to feel guilty or upset if a dose is forgotten or the wrong insulin given, but try not to, as in most cases adjustments can be made and no ill effects will be had. Keep in mind that fluctuations are natural and blood glucose levels vary.

Treatment of type 2 diabetes

The mainstay of treatment for type 2 diabetes is diet and lifestyle changes. This involves the whole family. It is very difficult to change the diet and habits of one child without affecting all family members. In any case, everyone, with or without diabetes, should be eating healthily and taking exercise. This helps prevent obesity and may also prevent others in the family from developing type 2 diabetes.

Your dietician can advise you on a healthy diet that will help with weight loss if needed, but will also give good control of blood glucose levels (see Chapter 6, 'Diet and staying well'). Although type 2 diabetes is associated with being overweight, children should not be placed on a very restrictive, extremely low calorie diet to help them lose weight. Rather, a healthy eating plan should be started, with an increase in exercise. This leads to a slow weight loss but is easier to manage than a very restrictive diet.

Exercise can be anything that your child enjoys that also gets his heart rate up. Start slowly; it is disheartening to set huge targets and then not be able to reach them. Set small, achievable goals. Try to be active in some way every day, for at least 30 minutes. This can mean anything from walking to school instead of driving, or getting off the bus one or two stops early and walking the rest of the way, to a dance or martial arts class, rollerblading, swimming, going out on a bike or just kicking a ball around with friends. You could get the whole family involved, going on country walks or bike rides. You may find your child learns a new skill or makes new friends at the same time.

It may be that diet and lifestyle changes alone do not control blood glucose levels. Medications may then be started. Starting medication does not mean that you can stop eating a healthy diet, the medications are used together with lifestyle changes. If necessary; combinations of medications can be used.

- *Metformin* This is generally the first medication used. This works to decrease insulin resistance so the cells can use the glucose in the blood. It also stops the liver from producing more glucose from its stores of glycogen. It only works if some insulin is still being produced by the pancreas. It can also help overweight people lose weight. It does not cause hypoglycaemia. There may be side effects such as feeling sick and tummy pain, but these generally go away with time.
- *Sulphonylureas* This is a group of medication that includes the tablets gliclazide and glibenclamide. They help boost the amount of insulin secreted by the pancreas.
- *Insulin treatment* This is often not needed in type 2 diabetes. However with time, there is a chance that the pancreas may stop secreting insulin. If insulin treatment is required, it is exactly the same as for type 1 diabetes. Even with well-controlled type 2 diabetes, an insulin drip may be needed during an operation or a medical emergency.

Children with type 2 diabetes will be seen regularly by the diabetes team and screened for the long-term complications of diabetes (see Chapter 8, 'Long-term complications').

Common questions

- *How can I prevent my other children from getting type 2 diabetes?* Doctors are not exactly sure why diabetes occurs, but as type 2 diabetes is associated with being overweight, keeping weight within a healthy range should help prevent other children from developing type 2 diabetes.
- *My child has type 2 diabetes, does this mean he has to have insulin treatment?* Not necessarily. Most people with type 2 diabetes can control their blood glucose levels with a healthy diet and lifestyle changes such as increased exercise. If these changes are not sufficient, medications can be started.
- *Is my child at risk of hypoglycaemic attacks?* Hypoglycaemia occurs either because too little food has been eaten or too much insulin has been given. If you are controlling type 2 diabetes with diet and lifestyle changes, you are not at risk of developing hypoglycaemia. Metformin also does not cause hypoglycaemia; however, the sulphonylurea group of medicines and insulin treatment can cause hypoglycaemia.

6

Diet and staying well

The word 'diet' refers to what food we eat and does not necessarily mean that you are trying to lose weight. There is no real difference between a 'healthy diet' and a 'diabetic diet'. After all, no one, whether or not they have diabetes, should be eating lots of chocolate and junk food every day! The whole family should eat a healthy diet. This makes it easier for the person preparing the food as well as for the people eating it! Your family will quickly adjust if you only have healthy food around. A healthy diet does not mean that you only eat the things that are 'good' for you. It means eating a wide variety of different things and occasionally allowing yourself treats. And, in diabetes, a healthy diet helps control blood glucose levels.

Remember, having diabetes does not mean that people cannot eat carbohydrates or sugary foods. There are times, such as during a hypoglycaemic episode, when eating something sugary is necessary.

The aims of this chapter are to discuss the components of a healthy diet and how different food types are absorbed by the body. The dietician in your diabetes team will also be able to give you advice on diet and meal planning. Methods of calculating how much insulin is needed depending on what you have eaten, such as carbohydrate counting, will be discussed as will the differing nutritional needs of your child at various ages.

Glycaemic index

The body needs glucose for energy. We obtain glucose from the carbohydrates in food. Enzymes in saliva and acids and enzymes in the stomach all help to break the carbohydrates down into glucose. Once the glucose has entered the small intestine, it is absorbed into the bloodstream for use by the body's cells. Various factors affect how quickly the food can be broken down and therefore be used.

The glycaemic index (GI) refers to how quickly a food can be broken down and used by the body, i.e. how quickly a food causes a rise in blood glucose level. Food with a high glycaemic index causes a rapid increase in blood glucose levels. This is generally followed by a rapid fall in blood glucose levels which may cause hunger or even hypogly-caemia. Pure glucose has the highest glycaemic index. Food with a low GI does not cause a rapid rise in blood glucose; it takes longer to be broken down into simple sugars and therefore to be absorbed by the body. Low GI foods result in a slow steady release of glucose into the bloodstream, providing the body with a constant, steady source of energy. All carbohydrates affect blood glucose levels. However, you can influence the glycaemic index of meals by changing what you eat and how food is prepared.

Examples of high glycaemic-index foods include processed white bread, cakes and sweets. The body does not have to work very hard to break down these foods into their simple sugars. How the food is prepared also has an effect. Bread and pasta are both made from wheat; however, pasta has a lower glycaemic index than bread. Preparation methods that break down the food, even before you eat it, increase the glycaemic index, such as mashing a potato in comparison to boiling it, or juicing an apple. The body absorbs fluids quickly, so soup or juice lead to a quicker rise in blood sugar than bread. Drinking lots of fluids with your meal helps the stomach empty quickly so the glucose enters the intestine quickly, raising blood glucose levels. If your blood glucose levels are low, your stomach empties more quickly than if blood glucose levels are high, as the body attempts to correct the hypoglycaemia.

Low glycaemic-index foods include complex carbohydrates that take the body a long time to break down, such as granary breads, or beans, nuts and vegetables. Cooking foods such as beans or lentils does not affect their structure, so the body still has to work to break them down itself. Foods that are high in fibre (such as fruit and vegetables) or have some fat content (from meat or dairy) make you feel fuller for longer and also stop the stomach from emptying too quickly into the small intestine. This means that the stomach releases a slow steady stream of food into the small intestine, resulting in a steady release of glucose. A chocolate bar contains some fat so has a lower glycaemic index than boiled sweets. Adding foods that contain fibre or fat to your meal decreases the glycaemic index of the meal.

How much you eat is also important. Although sweets have a high glycaemic index, eating only one sweet will not have a large effect on blood glucose levels as there is not a lot of glucose in only one sweet. The more you eat, even of a very low glycaemic-index food, the greater the effect it has on your blood glucose level. Because of this, treat foods can be eaten, as long as they are only eaten in small amounts as part of a healthy diet.

Understanding how the body digests different types of carbohydrate allows you to understand what you need in your diet. For example, if you know your child will be doing a lot of exercise, then a slow energy-releasing breakfast such as porridge is better than a high glycaemic-index breakfast such as a sugary cereal. It also helps you understand appropriate snacks. If you know that your child gets hypoglycaemic in the afternoon, then a snack such as a handful of dried fruit and nuts would be appropriate. The dried fruit acts quickly to raise the blood glucose levels, nuts have a low glycaemic index and should help to provide the body with glucose until your next meal. If the snack were simply sweets, although the blood glucose level rises, it also falls again quickly, so that your child needs to eat again. In a very severe hypoglycaemic episode, eating glucose tablets leads to a quicker rise in blood glucose than a chocolate bar (which contains fat) and so is a more appropriate choice, as long as it is followed up with a longer-acting carbohydrate such as a sandwich.

A 'healthy' diet

Perhaps one of the most important points is to eat! Your child should eat three meals a day, with healthy snacks if needed, and breakfast is indeed the most important meal of the day. It is not a good idea to miss meals, especially with diabetes, as it increases the risk of hypoglycaemia. Your diet should be based around the major food groups: carbohydrates, protein and fats.

Carbohydrates

Carbohydrates include cereals, breads, pasta, rice, certain vegetables such as potatoes and corn, fruit, milk, cakes, biscuits, chocolate and sweets. Base each meal around a starchy carbohydrate to give a slow steady release of energy. Examples include porridge or muesli for breakfast, granary bread in lunch sandwiches, and brown pasta or rice with your evening meal. Try and limit simple sugars such as sweets that cause a short sharp rise in blood glucose levels. Sugary foods also cause problems with tooth decay and are often high in calories, so may cause weight problems.

Protein

Protein is needed to provide material for the body to build new cells and tissues. Proteins include meat, poultry, fish, eggs, nuts and beans and should make up about a fifth of each meal. Protein does not contain any glucose so will not have a direct effect on blood sugar levels and therefore cannot be used to treat or prevent hypoglycaemia. Again, some protein is healthier than others. This depends on how much fat the food also contains. For example, a portion of chicken without the skin on contains much less fat than a steak.

Fish, especially oily fish, is important, as it contains vitamins and minerals and fats that keep the heart healthy. Currently the recommendation is to eat at least two portions of fish each week, including one portion of oily fish such as salmon. Fish that is fresh, or has been frozen or smoked, all count towards your portion of fish.

Fats

Many people think that fat is bad for you. However, you need some fat in your diet to stay healthy. There are different types of fat: saturated fat such as that in butter and processed meats and sausages, and unsaturated fat such as that found in nuts, avocados and olive oil. Eating too much saturated fat increases the risk of developing high cholesterol and increases the risk of developing heart disease. One of the long-term complications of diabetes is heart disease, so it is advisable to try to reduce the amount of saturated fat and instead include unsaturated fats. Fats are high in calories and so eating too much fat may cause weight gain. About one-eighth of your meals should be from foods that contain fats.

So, try to avoid too many sausages, pastries, biscuits or butter as these contain saturated fats. Some foods such as red meat are high in saturated fat but are also a good source of protein, so they can be included occasionally. Try healthy fats such as those found in nuts.

Fruit and vegetables

We should aim to eat at least five portions of fruit and vegetables every day. Fruit and vegetables contain fibre and vitamins and minerals vital to the body. Fruit and vegetables can be fresh, frozen, dried, tinned or juiced and still count towards your five portions a day. About a third of each meal should be made up of fruit and vegetables.

Try fruit juice and an apple or banana with breakfast, carrot sticks with lunch, cooked or raw vegetables with dinner and fruit as snacks.

Most vegetables do not have much effect on blood sugar. They are also low in calories, so your child (and you!) can eat a lot of them without worrying about putting on weight. However, potatoes, beans and sweet corn do contain carbohydrates and therefore affect blood glucose. Fruit contains carbohydrates and the fruit sugar fructose. It is absorbed quickly by the body, so a fruit juice is a good source of sugar during a hypoglycaemic episode.

Fibre

Fibre is needed to prevent constipation. It also makes food bulky and so fills up your stomach, making you feel full. There are two types of fibre: insoluble and soluble. The body cannot absorb insoluble fibre, such as that found in bran. This fibre adds bulk to your stools and helps stop you getting constipated. Soluble fibre also helps prevent constipation, and has an effect on blood glucose. Soluble fibre is found in fruit and vegetables.

Water

Fluids stop the body getting dehydrated. The average person requires about eight large glasses or two litres of water per day. In diabetes, glucose may be excreted in the urine, and your child may be urinating very frequently. This means that he is losing a lot of water and is the reason why people with uncontrolled diabetes are often very thirsty. When blood glucose levels are high, people need to drink even more than the two litres of water recommended per day. If your child becomes dehydrated, you may notice that he complains of headaches, tiredness, problems concentrating, and passing very concentrated, strong urine.

Most fluids count towards your two litres per day, from water to juices to fizzy drinks. Remember though that fruit juices and non-diet soft drinks lead to a rise in blood glucose levels. Diet fizzy drinks contain artificial sweeteners instead of sugar and so do not have an effect on blood glucose levels. Milk is a good choice as it contains calcium and protein, though it also contains fat. Some drinks, such as tea, coffee or soft drinks such as Coca-Cola contain caffeine, which acts as a diuretic and so may lead to more frequent urination and even dehydration. Children should not have too much caffeine anyway as it can cause agitation, poor sleep, and appetite problems. Children should not drink alcohol.

Salt

Too much salt can increase blood pressure, a risk factor for developing heart disease. As this is a long-term complication of diabetes, salt should be limited. The recommended maximum amount of salt per day in children over 11 years old is 6 grams; children under 11 need much less. Do not add salt to food, cook with herbs instead of salt to give flavour and avoid eating lots of processed foods as these often contain high levels of salt.

Meals and snacks throughout your day should be balanced according to Figure 8. Do not forget to include drinks. Remember that some foods

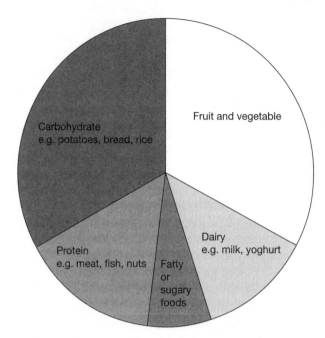

Figure 8 The 'perfect' plate – don't forget to include fluids!

overlap different food groups. For example, milk provides fluids, dairy, fat and protein; corn is a carbohydrate but also a vegetable; meat is a protein but also contains fat. A food like pizza contains a lot of carbohydrates from the bread base, but also dairy, fat and protein from the cheese and can have various vegetable, meat or fish toppings.

Food requirements at different ages

Children of different ages need differing amounts and types of food. Toddlers and very young children are growing very quickly and are very active so they need lots of energy from their food. They are also not able to eat a lot of food at a time so need to eat small amounts regularly. They should be eating a healthy diet, as described above. Children up to two years old should drink full fat milk to help provide them with calories for energy.

Children are generally quite good at telling you that they are full, as they stop eating. This is also true of children with diabetes, as long as their blood glucose levels are well controlled. You should not try and force them to finish their meal. Only healthy snacks should be offered in between meals. If blood glucose levels are high, your child may not feel hungry and so will eat less. Sometimes, if diabetes is not well controlled, hyperglycaemia may make your child feel hungry; for this reason it is important to check blood glucose levels regularly.

The speed at which your child grows slows down after early childhood until puberty. During the growth spurts of puberty children's energy and therefore food requirements increase. Again, they should follow the healthy diet described above. Once he has stopped growing, your child again needs to eat less. (See Chapter 10 on puberty and adolescence.)

Carbohydrate counting

Carbohydrates of any kind act to increase blood glucose levels. Insulin is then needed to help cells use the glucose so blood levels return to normal. Carbohydrate counting involves working out how much insulin is needed to counteract the carbohydrates in each meal. There are different methods of carbohydrate counting, and your dietician can teach you the method used in your team. A simple method involves using tables that list the amount of carbohydrates in food, for example, the average-sized baked potato. You can then give the relevant amount of insulin, but this is different for each child depending on factors such as their weight and previous blood glucose control. You will be advised how many grams of carbohydrate is covered by one unit of insulin. More complicated methods involve weighing up the amount of carbohydrates eaten against the amount of activity you are about to do to help decide the appropriate insulin dose.

Snacks

Whether or not your child has to have snacks depends on the insulin regime that you use. People without diabetes secrete very little insulin between meals. If you are using a basal bolus regimen you may not need a snack in between meals as the insulin regime is very close to that of someone without diabetes. If you are using a twice- or three-times-daily regime your child needs a snack to balance the effect of the intermediate- or long-acting insulin to prevent hypoglycaemia.

Snacks should provide a balance of quickly and slowly absorbed carbohydrates. The quickly absorbed carbohydrates bring blood glucose levels up quickly to prevent hypoglycaemia, the longer-acting carbohydrates prevent hypoglycaemia until the next meal.

Examples of healthy snacks include: fresh or dried fruit, nuts, cereal bars or bowl of cereal, oatcakes, low fat crisps, a piece of malt or fruit loaf, unsweetened yoghurt, or a sandwich such as peanut butter. See below for a recipe for a healthy snack.

Treats

Treats are part of everyone's diet. The key is to limit how often you eat them – after all, if you ate them daily, they would not be treats! Remember, even if your child did not have diabetes, you would probably still limit the amount of treats he was allowed. If you never allow your child treats and sweets he will probably still eat them anyway, without your knowledge, so his diabetes will not be managed appropriately.

Even if you do not have treats such as sweets and cakes at home, your child will see his or her friends eating them and may be offered them when playing or at parties. It is important that your child does not feel too different from his or her peers. Let him have treats occasionally. You can compensate for the rise in blood glucose with extra insulin or by having the treat instead of another carbohydrate within the same meal. Alternatively, you could give half a normal snack such as a sandwich, and replace the other half with a treat that contains the equivalent amount of carbohydrate. Even within treats some types have a quicker effect on blood glucose levels than others. You can give extra rapid-acting insulin for sweets, and short-acting insulin for treats that contain fat (and so take longer to cause a rise in blood glucose) such as chocolate or ice cream.

'Diabetic' food

If a foodstuff is marketed as 'diabetic', it does not necessarily mean that it is healthy. Lots of these foods are cakes, biscuits and chocolate bars that do not have as much sugar in them as ordinary cakes etc. However, in order to make them taste nice they may actually contain more fat and be higher in calories. Therefore, they may actually be worse for your health. Foods such as cakes should be considered treats, and not part of your everyday diet. These 'diabetic' foods are also often expensive.

Chewy oat, fruit and nut bars

These bars could be used as a snack food. The dried fruit and honey act quickly to increase the blood glucose levels, while the nuts and oats tide you over until the next meal.

Ingredients:

250 g plain oats
60 g margarine or butter
4 tablespoons of clear runny honey

250 g mixed unsweetened dried fruit and nuts. You can use any combination – try raisins, sultanas, chopped dried apricots, chopped dates, dried cranberries, dried blueberries, dried sour cherries, dried banana chips, any kind of nuts. Use unsweetened brands if possible.

- Preheat the oven to 180°C.
- In a saucepan, melt the margarine and honey together until they are liquid. Don't let the mixture boil. Take the mixture off the heat.
- Stir in the oats until they are well coated with the margarine and honey mixture.
- Add the mixed fruit and nuts and mix well.
- Pour the mixture onto a baking tray and spread it out evenly. Run a rolling pin over the top of the tray so the mixture lies flat.
- Bake in the oven until golden brown – approximately 12 minutes. If you like the bars crunchy instead of chewy, cook for approximately 15 minutes.
- Take out of the oven and leave to cool.
- Once cool cut into squares and store in an airtight container.

Diabetes and being unwell

Insulin requirements may change if your child is unwell, even with a relatively minor illness such as a cold with a temperature. This is related to the body's natural response to fight illness. It is common to assume that if a child is unwell and therefore not eating very much then he needs less insulin. This is not the case; when unwell, children may in fact need even more insulin to prevent hyperglycaemia and potentially diabetic ketoacidosis.

Having a temperature

A temperature is one of the body's defence mechanisms against the virus or bacteria causing an infection such as a cold, which may not be able to survive in the hotter environment. Increased amounts of the stress hormone cortisol are secreted. One of the actions of cortisol is to increase blood glucose levels. In those without diabetes, the pancreas automatically secretes more insulin to counteract the effects of the glucose-raising hormones.

Therefore, if a child has any kind of infection, he needs more insulin to prevent hyperglycaemia. However, generally, if children have a fever or are unwell they tend to eat less. The need for more insulin has to be balanced against the fact that they are eating less – as always, giving too much insulin can lead to hypoglycaemia. It is recommended that the normal amount of insulin be given during the day, but that you check blood glucose levels and urine for ketones regularly, in case you need to increase insulin doses. Try to provide regular snacks that involve carbohydrates. Do not forget to encourage your child to drink lots of fluids and take paracetamol (the sugar-free formulas!) to decrease any temperature.

Vomiting and gastroenteritis

Children, especially young children, may vomit whenever they have a temperature or any infection. Vomiting can also be a sign of an infection in the stomach or digestive system; if vomiting occurs with diarrhoea it is called gastroenteritis. As with any infection, insulin requirements go up in illness.

It is important to remember that feeling sick, nauseous or vomiting is also a sign of insulin deficiency and ketoacidosis. Hypoglycaemia may also make a person feel sick. If your child starts vomiting always check blood glucose levels and urine for ketones. High blood glucose levels and urinary ketones indicate insulin deficiency. Low blood glucose levels and urinary ketones indicate that not enough food has been eaten (starvation ketones).

You need to give insulin but also glucose to prevent hypoglycaemia. If vomiting, a child may not be able to tolerate meals or even a large drink. Give small amounts of sugary drinks such as juices, or small snacks very regularly. If your child has diarrhoea and vomiting he may not be absorbing very much glucose from the food and drink, and insulin doses have to be decreased. Take blood glucose levels and urine tests regularly and adjust insulin and snacks as appropriate.

You should go to hospital if your child is vomiting so regularly that he is becoming dehydrated, if his temperature cannot be controlled with regular paracetamol, or if his blood glucose levels or urinary ketones remain high or rising despite insulin, or if he has a hypoglycaemic episode that you cannot correct at home. He may need continuous treatment with insulin and glucose through a drip.

Having an operation

Having any operation, even a small one such as having a tooth removed, causes stress to the body and so may increase insulin requirements. You should always inform any doctor or dentist that your child has diabetes.

If your child is having a general anaesthetic he will be asked not to eat for at least six hours before the operation. This can cause problems for people with diabetes, so he will generally be put first on the operating list in the morning.

Immunizations

Children with diabetes should be vaccinated according to the national immunization programme. The Department of Health also currently recommends that children with diabetes who are over six months old should also be vaccinated against influenza every year. This vaccination is available, free of charge, from your GP.

Common questions

- *My child has a sore throat and a temperature and does not want to eat. How much insulin should I give?* Start by giving the same amount of insulin as normal. Your child needs more insulin due to the effects of the illness but this should be balanced against the fact that he is eating less, so giving the normal amount of insulin is a good starting point. Test blood glucose regularly and adjust insulin doses if required. Give regular snacks and lots of fluids.

- *Should I give more or less insulin when my child is vomiting?* You need to check blood glucose levels and urinary ketones before deciding how much insulin to give. Vomiting can be a sign of infection or a sign of insulin deficiency. If blood glucose levels are high and there are urinary ketones, more insulin is needed as this indicates insulin deficiency. If blood glucose levels are low and there are ketones in the urine, then it is likely that the vomiting is caused by an infection and your child is not absorbing enough glucose from her food (before vomiting it back up). If so, you should give very regular sugary snacks such as fruit juice and could decrease the insulin dose to prevent hypoglycaemia. Check blood glucose levels and urinary ketones very regularly.

- *When should you go to hospital?* You can contact your diabetes team whenever you need help; if they are not available, you can always go to your local hospital if you feel that you are not managing. You should also go to hospital if blood glucose levels are rising or if your child still has ketones after having extra insulin, or if your child becomes very unwell with high blood glucose levels. If your child is vomiting so regularly or continuously that he is becoming dehydrated or if his temperature does not return to normal with regular paracetamol you should also go to the hospital. Do not ever think that your child is not unwell enough to see a doctor. If you are worried and do not feel that you can control his diabetes while he is unwell, then you should seek advice and go to hospital.

7

Diabetic emergencies: hypoglycaemia and hyperglycaemia

Hypoglycaemia

Hypoglycaemia is the medical term for low levels of blood glucose, which may make people feel unwell. Generally, either the person eats more, or the body releases more glucose from its stores to bring the levels back up to normal. If however the levels get extremely low there is a risk of having fits and losing consciousness, as the brain needs glucose to function properly. Therefore it is important to be able to recognize the symptoms of hypoglycaemia at an early stage when it can be easily treated. It is currently not clear what, if any, effect recurrent hypoglycaemia has on the brain.

What are the symptoms of hypoglycaemia?

Not everyone gets the same symptoms at the same blood glucose levels. Some people are more sensitive, or are more aware of their symptoms at a higher blood glucose level than others. The body secretes hormones such as adrenaline to increase the blood glucose, and the adrenaline causes some of the symptoms of hypoglycaemia such as feeling shaky (autonomic or adrenergic symptoms). Other symptoms are related to the effects of the low blood glucose on the brain, preventing it from working properly (neuroglycopenic symptoms).

Symptoms include:

- feeling hungry or sick;
- looking pale;
- feeling your heart pounding;
- shakiness and trembling;
- feeling sweaty, cold and clammy;
- feeling very hot;
- feeling anxious;
- getting irritable and snappy;
- numbness or pins and needles feeling in your lips and fingers;
- feeling weak;

- feeling dizzy;
- behaving oddly;
- problems with concentrating;
- being confused, or having difficulty remembering things;
- blurring or double vision;
- problems with hearing, such as everything becoming muffled or sounding far away;
- headaches;
- feeling tired or drowsy;
- difficulties with speech such as slurred speech;
- problems with walking or co-ordination;
- fits (seizures);
- loss of consciousness.

Not everyone gets all these symptoms. The list is long and scary, but remember that it includes the symptoms of the dangerously low, potentially life-threatening levels of hypoglycaemia as well as the more common symptoms of an easily treatable hyperglycaemia. Seizures tend not to occur until the blood glucose level is close to 1 mmol/l.

The body reacts to hypoglycaemia by first producing the hormones that bring up the blood glucose level. These hormones produce the autonomic symptoms so you are more likely to get these symptoms first. These include looking pale, feeling clammy and the heart pounding. The brain does not produce symptoms (such as problems concentrating or drowsiness) until the blood sugar is at a lower level, so there is the opportunity to do something about the hypoglycaemia, i.e. get food, while one is able. The lower the blood sugar, the less able the brain is to help make decisions and therefore the less able one becomes to help oneself. This is why it is important that you, your child, or someone else is able to recognize the symptoms of hypoglycaemia at an early stage.

Children are more likely to experience behavioural changes than adults when hypoglycaemic. You may notice that your child becomes pale and sweaty but also gets argumentative or tearful. She may not be able to express how she feels, so it may come across as naughtiness or clinginess.

How well the child herself recognizes the symptoms of hypoglycaemia depends on how accustomed she is to the symptoms or whether or not she is concentrating hard on something else. It also depends on recent blood glucose levels. If they have been higher than normal, symptoms are experienced at a higher blood glucose level, sometimes when the blood sugar is still within the normal range. This is because if blood glucose level was about 7 mmol/l for the preceding few days, a drop to 5 mmol/l will be recognized by the body as significant. Conversely, if in the past few days blood glucose level has been low, the body adjusts to this and does not produce symptoms until a much lower blood glucose level, for example if glucose was 4.5 mmol/l for a few days, one may not develop symptoms until a level of 3 mmol/l. Finally, some children get symptoms of hypoglycaemia even when their blood glucose is high. It can be difficult to distinguish the symptoms of hypoglycaemia and hyperglycaemia. This is because in diabetes, when there is hyperglycaemia, the cells react as in starvation, as they do not have insulin to allow glucose to enter the cells. It can be difficult, especially in young children, to differentiate between hunger from hypoglycaemia and the reaction of the body to hyperglycaemia. Checking the blood glucose level tells you which is occurring.

When should I check blood glucose for hypoglycaemia?

You should check your blood glucose whenever your child feels unwell, strange, or has any of the symptoms described above. Initially, you may feel you are checking for hypoglycaemia very often, especially as treatment is being adjusted. However, it is better to check more times than perhaps needed so that you do not miss a hypoglycaemic episode, as these need to be treated. With time, you may be better at recognizing your child's particular set of symptoms of hypoglycaemia.

What blood glucose level is hypoglycaemia?

If the 'normal' blood glucose range is between about 4.0 and 6.5 mmol/l, you can consider anything less than about 4 mmol/l to be hypoglycaemia. In people without diabetes, the symptoms of hypoglycaemia develop at a glucose level of approximately 3 mmol/l. As mentioned above, the level at which you develop the symptoms of hypoglycaemia depends on your normal average blood glucose levels. If you have a high HbA1c you may develop symptoms at a higher blood glucose level than if you have a very low HbA1c.

Remember, if your blood glucose machine reads 'low', do not assume that it is an incorrect reading. Some machines stop reading once the blood glucose is below a certain level and just say 'low'. If your machine says 'low' and your child is feeling unwell, you should treat as for hypoglycaemia.

Why does hypoglycaemia occur?

Hypoglycaemia occurs because either not enough food has been eaten, or too much insulin has been used. Reasons for not having enough food include missing a snack or a meal, doing more physical exercise than normal, or being unwell with vomiting or diarrhoea. Alternatively you may have used a new site for injection so the insulin is absorbed quicker than expected. If your child has already had a recent hypoglycaemic episode she may have used up her glycogen stores and so is more susceptible to further episodes.

What should I do?

The treatment of hypoglycaemia is to give glucose! Everyone involved with someone with diabetes needs to know how to help when hypoglycaemia occurs – the person affected, his or her parents and family, schoolteachers and friends. Don't go out without a supply of glucose tablets or gel or a snack or carton of juice. If your child is going on a school trip or overnight camping, she should always take glucagon (see below). Many people have a misconception that people with diabetes cannot have anything sugary and so won't give the sugar needed unless you have taught them otherwise.

Glucose in any form, from pure sugar to a complex carbohydrate, can be used to bring up the blood glucose. Remember, though, that the body can only absorb glucose once the food is in the small intestine. So, if you need to bring the blood glucose level up quickly you need to use a simple sugar; to bring it up slower over a longer period of time a more complex carbohydrate can be used. A glucose drink such as Lucozade, or glucose tablets, work in about 15 minutes, a bar of chocolate takes about 30 minutes.

There are various methods of giving glucose depending on the degree of hypoglycaemia and how well the child is and therefore how able she is to take the glucose.

If your child feels unwell, you should always test blood sugar as the symptoms may not necessarily be caused by hypoglycaemia. If, however, blood sugar levels are low, your child should eat something sweet, like a glucose tablet, or drink an energy drink containing glucose. It is better not to overcompensate by eating too much sugar, to avoid blood glucose levels becoming too high. Start small and then if there is no improvement in about 15 minutes, take the blood sugar again and eat a bit more. The amount your child needs to eat depends on her weight. The average glucose tablet contains about 3 g of glucose; this brings up the blood glucose of a 20 kg child by 2 mmol/l. Also, any exercise should stop as it worsens the hypoglycaemia.

Your child may find it difficult to eat; after all, the brain is not functioning quite as well as it should. Gels that contain glucose such as GlucoGel (previously called HypoStop), or honey or jam, may be easier to swallow.

Glucagon

If the child is more unwell, or even unconscious, then she may need an injection of glucagon. Glucagon can be seen as the opposite hormone to insulin. It is released when blood sugar levels are low and helps the body release its stores of glucose from the glycogen in the liver and produce glucose from proteins and fats as well as stimulating ketone production. Giving an injection of glucagon helps these processes to occur and hopefully bring up the blood glucose levels.

Glucagon is given by an injection just under the skin (for more on giving injections see Chapter 4). The dose of glucagon is 0.1–0.2 mg per 10 kg of body weight. Therefore if your child weighs 25 kg, you need to give 0.25–0.5 mg of glucagon. Do not worry about giving too much glucagon by mistake as it is not dangerous. The injection takes about 15 minutes to work and then lasts for between 30 minutes and an hour, which should give time to eat something. As the glucagon injection stimulates the production of ketones it might make your child feel sick, so she should try and wait about half an hour before eating.

Glucagon injections do not always work. This may be because the glycogen stores have already been used up, for example in exercise, or they have not had a chance to be built back up from recent hypoglycaemic attacks. Alternatively the effects of the glucagon might be cancelled out if too much insulin has been given. In these situations, giving a second dose may not have an effect and is likely to make the person feel sick or even vomit, which may worsen the situation.

The glucagon injection may have to be mixed before you can give it. In this kind of situation you may find it difficult to stay calm, so practise how you would draw up the glucagon and set up to give an injection beforehand.

What if the treatment does not work?

If glucagon does not work, or if the child is unconscious despite normal blood glucose levels, call an ambulance. She may need treatment in hospital with continuous glucose into the veins by a drip (or in the worst-case scenario have swelling in the brain that needs observation and treatment). It is better to be cautious than to leave a severe hypoglycaemia untreated.

Instructions for treating hypoglycaemia

- If possible, test the blood glucose. If not possible and the child has symptoms, treat as for hypoglycaemia.

- If the level is below 3.5 mmol/l at any time or between 3.5 and 4.5 mmol/l and the next meal is over half an hour away, give glucose.
- The glucose can be in the form of anything such as glucose tablets or drink, a carton of juice or fizzy drink or even simple sugar!
- If the child is finding it difficult to chew, consider a drink like Lucozade or glucose gel such as GlucoGel (previously called HypoStop).
- If he becomes unconscious or has severe hypoglycaemia consider giving an injection of glucagon.
- If he does not improve, or remains unconscious, call an ambulance.
- If he does improve, he may need to eat something to tide him over until the next meal to prevent another episode of hypoglycaemia.

What happens after an episode of hypoglycaemia?

Once the hypoglycaemia is treated and blood glucose levels have returned to normal your child should feel better very quickly. However, it might take a few hours for the body to recover fully so that she is back at her best. She may get headaches. You need to think how long it is until the next proper meal and therefore how much she will need to eat in the meantime to prevent another episode of hypoglycaemia. No matter how long the gap until the next meal, your child should wait 15 minutes after taking a glucose tablet or sugary drink before eating to allow time for it to be absorbed. If she eats straight away, the food will mix with the glucose in the stomach and prevent the glucose tablet or drink from being absorbed quickly. If it is less than an hour before the next meal, she may need something small like some fruit to tide her over; if it is a few hours, something more substantial like a sandwich may be needed.

Rebound phenomenon

During the episode of hypoglycaemia, the body tries to correct the levels of blood glucose itself by the production of the various regulatory hormones such as glucagon and adrenaline. People also feel hungry and may eat more than they need. The rebound phenomenon is when blood glucose becomes higher than normal in the period after hypoglycaemia, due to the effects of these hormones and the extra food. This only occurs if someone does not have enough insulin in the blood to counteract these hormones during this time, so do not decrease the insulin dose before the next meal in an attempt to prevent hypoglycaemia occurring again.

Hypoglycaemia at night

It is very common to become hypoglycaemic at night and people may not be woken up by the symptoms. Regular morning headaches, or having nightmares may be signs of night-time hypoglycaemia. The only way of knowing if a child gets night-time hypoglycaemia is to wake her up and test the blood glucose, about every couple of weeks. The rebound phenomenon may mean that in the morning her blood sugar is actually high and so you may think she needs more insulin at night, which will worsen the situation.

Hypoglycaemia at night can be caused by giving too much insulin before bed, not eating enough at the evening meal or a night-time snack. You could try changing the insulin dose or changing the bedtime snack to a slow-releasing carbohydrate such as granary bread or corn-starch bar to ensure that the glucose is released steadily during the night. If your child's pre-bed blood glucose level is in the lower range of normal, get her to eat something extra.

Recognizing hypoglycaemia

If your child feels unwell and her blood glucose is low, try to recall the symptom that made you take the test. If you can work out what your child's symptoms of hypoglycaemia are, you will become more aware of them and may be able to recognize the development of hypoglycaemia.

Hypoglycaemia unawareness

This means people have low blood glucose without any autonomic 'warning' symptoms, and can occur if they normally have blood glucose levels at the lower range of normal or if they regularly have hypoglycaemic episodes. It can also occur when they have had diabetes for many years as the body may start to release less adrenaline when the blood glucose levels are low. As the adrenaline is responsible for the autonomic symptoms such as going pale and feeling shaky, some people do not have any triggering symptoms and can develop hypoglycaemia unawareness. This leads to an increased risk of developing severe hypoglycaemia as without symptoms, the person may not recognize the low blood glucose levels at a time when this can be easily treated.

If you are aware that your child has hypoglycaemia unawareness you need to try and reset her hypoglycaemia body clock. Avoid having low blood sugars for a couple of weeks, even if this means accepting higher blood glucose levels than you would like. With time, the body's response to hypoglycaemia will reset and she will develop the symptoms of hypoglycaemia at a higher level than previously, allowing you to treat the low blood glucose appropriately.

Hyperglycaemia and diabetic ketoacidosis

Hyperglycaemia is the term for blood glucose levels higher than the normal range, i.e. above 7 mmol/l prior to a meal. The body tries to excrete the high levels of blood glucose into the urine. There may or may not be symptoms relating to hyperglycaemia (see below). The only way of knowing may be to check with a blood glucose monitor.

If blood glucose levels are high due to insulin deficiency, the cells cannot access the high levels of glucose, and so respond as if they were starving. The body acts to try to release as much glucose as possible in order to keep working, without realizing that there are already high levels of glucose in the blood. So the body releases more glucose, from glycogen in the liver, and by breaking down proteins, for example from the muscles. Fat stores are also used to release glucose, the components of fat are broken down into glycerol and free fatty acids. The glycerol is then converted into glucose and the free fatty acids into ketones. Ketones can be used instead of glucose as fuel for the brain. But, as there is still no insulin, the cells simply cannot access the glucose, and so the situation continues to spiral, the levels of blood glucose continue to rise, as does the production of ketones.

Ketones are significant as they make the blood more acidic than usual, which can affect the entire body. In the same way that the body can only function in a narrow range of temperatures, with the correct amount of water and blood glucose, the body can only work when at a certain level of acidity. How acid something is, is described by its pH: a low pH means something is acidic, and a high pH that it is alkaline (the opposite of acidic). The body works best when it has an almost neutral pH.

Possible symptoms of hyperglycaemia

- going to the toilet more regularly to pass urine, even at night (polyuria)
- being thirsty (polydypsia)

- dry mouth and skin from dehydration from passing urine so frequently
- skin itchiness or itching in the genitals
- tiredness
- blurred vision

The blurred vision of hyperglycaemia is not the same as the long-term eye complications of diabetes (see Chapter 8, 'Complications and associated conditions'). As the levels of glucose in the cells of the lens increase, the cells also try to absorb water so the lens swells. This swelling changes the shape of the lens in the eyes and vision may become blurred, in the same way as if the shape of the lenses in a pair of glasses were changed. As blood glucose levels return to normal, so does vision.

Symptoms of diabetic ketoacidosis

- feeling generally unwell and/or tired
- nausea and vomiting
- pain in the tummy or chest
- very sweet smell on your breath (described as the smell of pear drops)
- very deep heavy breathing, or problems with breathing
- weakness
- if the situation worsens, becoming drowsy or sleepy, eventually resulting in a coma – loss of consciousness

Remember, with increasing blood glucose levels, more glucose is excreted along with more fluid so people become thirsty and need to drink more to prevent dehydration. If a person becomes unable to drink he may become unwell very quickly, as fluid is needed to try to get rid of the ketones. Without drinking, levels can rise quickly. Vomiting is very often the first sign of insulin deficiency and ketoacidosis. It may be that your child simply has a tummy bug, but do the checks described below or contact your diabetes team, or go to your doctor.

Why does it occur and how can it be prevented?

Hyperglycaemia and ketoacidosis occur due to insulin deficiency as described above, and only in type 1 diabetes. As this is due to insulin deficiency, it can occur in any situation in which there is not enough insulin, for example if you forget to give an injection. It commonly occurs when more insulin than usual is needed, for example during puberty or illness. (See Chapter 5, 'Treatment of diabetes'.)

Ketoacidosis is also more likely if you use regular injections of rapid- or short-acting insulins, or an insulin pump, and do not use an intermediate- or long-acting 'basal'-type insulin. There is no store of insulin in the body as there would be with a longer-acting type of insulin, thus creating an increased risk of ketoacidosis.

Ketoacidosis does not always develop with hyperglycaemia. As long as there is some insulin, the cells have access to some of the glucose within the blood and therefore will not start the process that leads to ketoacidosis. Therefore it is not possible to predict a blood glucose level at which ketoacidosis will occur.

Hyperglycaemia and diabetic ketoacidosis are prevented by good control of blood glucose levels.

What tests can I do?

Testing blood glucose tells you if your child is hyperglycaemic, and a urine test tells you if she is also ketoacidotic. If there is glucose in the urine but no ketones, then she simply has hyperglycaemia; if there is both glucose and ketones in her urine then she has ketoacidosis.

How do you manage hyperglycaemia and ketoacidosis?

If your child has a one-off high blood glucose reading without ketones or feeling unwell she simply has hyperglycaemia, which can be treated with extra insulin depending on how close the next insulin dose is. For example, if hyperglycaemia occurs in the early afternoon and the next meal and insulin dose are not due for a few hours, you could consider a very small dose of rapid- or short-acting insulin to tide her over until the next dose. If hyperglycaemia occurs immediately before a meal, you could consider increasing the pre-meal insulin dose.

A person who has hyperglycaemia and ketones in her blood or urine is insulin deficient. Therefore you should give some extra short- or rapid-acting insulin. If, after a couple of hours blood glucose level remains high or has increased, or if she still has ketones in her blood, or increasing amounts of ketones in her urine, or becomes unwell at any stage, she needs to go to hospital for further treatment.

The hospital treatment for diabetic ketoacidosis involves an insulin drip, containing rapid-acting insulin at an appropriate level, and a second drip containing fluid with the correct amount of salts in it, such as potassium. There will also be regular blood and urine tests, as well as investigations for any cause such as an infection. Treatment is over a period of hours or days as it is not advisable to bring the blood glucose level down too quickly; it is done slowly to prevent other complications.

Hyper-osmolar non ketotic coma

Hyper-osmolar non ketotic coma (HONK) is the condition relating to severe hyperglycaemia in type 2 diabetes. In this case no ketones are produced but high blood glucose levels and dehydration result in lethargy and eventually coma. It is not common and is treated in hospital with intravenous fluids.

8

Long-term complications of diabetes and associated conditions

It is very common to be aware and fearful of the potential long-term complications of diabetes. People say things like, 'If you have diabetes you will go blind', or 'You will end up with kidney failure on dialysis', or 'having toes amputated'. Thankfully, we are much better at looking after diabetes now than we were years ago and different types of insulin and treatment regimes have been developed. Good control of blood glucose levels decreases the risk of developing complications, so diabetes should be controlled as tightly as possible without developing regular severe hypoglycaemic episodes.

It is unlikely that your child or teenager will be at the stage of suffering complications. However, it is important to learn about the potential complications, so you can do your best to prevent them occurring in later life. It is also important to be well informed so that neither you nor your child will be scared by rumours or exaggerated stories.

Diabetes has both short- and long-term complications and is a risk factor for developing other conditions.

Why do long-term complications occur?

It is currently not known exactly why long-term complications occur, or why they occur in certain people and not others. What is known is that the likelihood of complications is related to high blood glucose levels (and therefore high HbA1c levels) over time. The risk of complications also increases with the length of time that someone has had diabetes.

Most cells in the body cannot respond to glucose in the blood unless insulin is also present. However, certain cells can take glucose from the bloodstream and use it without insulin and can be damaged by high glucose levels. These include cells in the brain and nervous system, kidneys, in the walls of blood vessels, in the retina of the eye and red blood cells. Therefore, in these cells, the concentration of glucose in the cells is related to the concentration of glucose in the blood. When blood glucose levels are high, the concentration of glucose within these cells also becomes high.

This occurs because, even without diabetes, there are times when insulin production is turned off or decreased to almost nothing, such as during starvation. In this situation, only the most essential parts of the body – such as the brain – are able to use the limited supply of glucose in the blood without the need for insulin. This enables the body to continue to function in times of starvation.

In diabetes, unless insulin is injected, the blood glucose level rises, and continues to rise as the body tries to increase glucose levels even further. The high levels of glucose cause high levels of glucose in the particular cells that do not need insulin, and the glucose binds with other substances and causes damage. It is thought that it is this damage that causes the long-term complications of diabetes.

Complications do *not* occur directly because of eating sweets or cakes. Sweets themselves do not cause diabetic complications; they are caused by long-term high blood glucose levels due to poor diabetes control.

Complications in small blood vessels

Cells in the walls of blood vessels (tubes that carry blood through the body) can use glucose without needing insulin. After long periods of high blood glucose, glucose builds up in the cells of the vessel wall making vessels stiff. Glucose also builds up in the red blood cells in the blood, also making them stiff, so they cannot bend easily to fit through the tiniest of blood vessels (capillaries). Here, the tissues that these vessels supply may not get the oxygen that they need to function.

Nerves: diabetic neuropathy

The medical term for diabetic complications affecting nerves is 'diabetic neuropathy'. The nervous system is a system of lots of very long thin fibres made up of nerve cells, and is divided into two parts – the autonomic and the somatic nervous systems. The autonomic nervous system controls things such as your heart rate, blood pressure, digestive system and urinary system without you having to think about it. The somatic system conveys information from the skin to the brain, such as temperature, touch or pain.

Both these systems can be affected in diabetes. Damage to the nerves is caused by the direct effect of high levels of glucose on the nerves, but also due to a decreased oxygen supply to the nerves from damaged small blood vessels. Long nerves are the most at risk. Nerves are covered in a sheath that helps transmit impulses along the nerve; this sheath is damaged and the speed of impulses slows down. With decreased sensation, the risk of infection increases as you may not notice and treat an injury.

Symptoms

Sensory neuropathy affects the nerves that carry sensation such as touch or vibration sense. As long nerves are affected first, you are most likely to get symptoms in your toes and feet or in your fingers. If severe, this may then begin to spread up the body. The nerves that carry the sensation of touch are affected first so you may have less sensation, or numbness, in these areas, or may develop tingling or 'pins and needles'. Pain sensation may also be decreased. This means that if you cut yourself or stand on something you may not feel it and so there is a risk of infection as you may not be aware of the injury. This is most likely in the feet: diabetes can cause feet to sweat less than normal and so the skin on your feet can become very dry and cracked, which can lead to ulcers forming.

Motor neuropathy is when the nerves of the motor system, which enable you to activate your muscles and therefore to move, are affected. It can cause muscle weakness.

The autonomic nervous system can also be affected (autonomic neuropathy), though this is less common. Symptoms include slow emptying of the stomach, constipation or diarrhoea, dizziness when standing up quickly or problems with emptying your bladder properly.

How is diabetic neuropathy prevented and treated?

Good diabetes control is the best treatment for neuropathy. If you think you are developing a neuropathy contact your doctor. As feet are the area most at risk of developing a loss of sensation, they are also most at risk of developing an infection. Therefore good foot hygiene and care are important. Feet should be cleaned as normal and checked for any cuts; toenails should be cut straight across. Your child should wear well-fitting shoes that do not cause blisters and not spend too much time barefoot as he may not be aware if he stands on something. Regular foot checks and care form part of your child's medical care.

Eyes: diabetic retinopathy

The retina is the area at the back of the eye where the light and images seen through the pupil are converted into nerve signals to be taken into the brain where they are converted back to an image so you can 'see'. The changes in diabetes affect the retina.

First tiny swellings can develop in the capillaries of the eyes as they become stiff and brittle with high levels of glucose. These are called microaneurysms and are not thought to cause any problems with vision. However, they can be considered as a warning sign. If blood glucose levels remain high, the changes can progress and worsen. The capillaries get so stiff they become blocked and the areas of the eye that they normally supply do not receive any oxygen or glucose. The eye then tries to grow more blood vessels to replace the blocked ones. These new capillaries are very fragile and very easily burst and bleed. Once new blood vessels are formed and there is repeated bleeding, damage to your vision may occur. In the early stages there are no symptoms and so you may not be aware that you are developing retinopathy.

Other eye problems that may occur in diabetes include an increased risk of developing cataracts (cloudiness of the lens of the eye that may need an operation) and glaucoma (increased pressure in the eye that is often treated with medication).

Blurred vision may also occur in hyperglycaemia or when blood glucose levels are changing rapidly, such as just after diagnosis. This blurred vision is not permanent (though it can last a few days or even a few weeks) and is not the same as diabetic retinopathy (see Chapter 7, 'Diabetic emergencies'). For this reason, eyes should only be tested when blood sugars are stable, otherwise you may find that your child's prescription needs changing!

How is diabetic retinopathy prevented and treated?

Good control of blood sugars can not only prevent retinopathy but even reverse the early changes of retinopathy. It is important that any changes are discovered early. In the UK, the National Institute for Health and Clinical Excellence (NICE) recommends an annual check for retinopathy from the age of 12.

The early changes of retinopathy do not require any treatment other than improving blood glucose control as much as possible. If new blood vessels start to develop in the eyes (proliferative retinopathy), this can be treated with laser treatment.

Kidneys: diabetic nephropathy

The role of the kidneys includes getting rid of waste products (urea) in the urine and keeping the correct balance of water and salts. If you are dehydrated, the kidneys preserve water for the body and you will not produce very much urine; what you do produce is very concentrated. Conversely, if you have too much water in the body, the kidneys produce a lot of weak urine in order to keep the water balance correct.

The small blood vessels in the kidneys can become damaged by long-term high blood glucose levels. The blood vessels become leaky and leak small amounts of protein into the urine, called microalbuminuria. If the damage worsens and the vessels become more leaky, more protein is released into the urine (proteinuria). Among other things this causes problems with high blood pressure. The kidneys stop being able to control the fluid balance in the body properly and swelling may develop, commonly in the ankles and feet. The body may also be unable to get rid of waste product urea, which in turn can cause problems. If the condition is not treated, kidney failure is a possibility.

How is diabetic nephropathy prevented and treated?

Again, good blood glucose control prevents the development of diabetic nephropathy and can even reverse the early stage of microalbuminuria. The current NICE guidelines are that children should be screened for microalbuminuria by a urine test every year, from the age of 12. If microalbuminuria does occur, oral medication with a class of drug called an ACE inhibitor (angiotensin-converting enzyme inhibitors, such as enalapril) is used. These medications are used in the control of high blood pressure, but are also beneficial for diabetic nephropathy even if your blood pressure is normal. Limiting the amount of protein in the diet should only be done if advised by your team, as protein is an essential part of the diet. Finally, if nephropathy is severe and cannot be treated with oral medication, dialysis may be started.

Complications in large blood vessels

Large blood vessels are also affected by long-term high blood glucose levels. They may become stiff and hard and can become narrowed by blockages, or even become blocked altogether (arteriosclerosis). Having diabetes increases the risk of developing arteriosclerosis. Other risk factors for arteriosclerosis include having high blood pressure, smoking, being overweight, having high levels of cholesterol and other fats in the blood and having a close family member with a history of heart problems. Arteriosclerosis and therefore diabetes increase the risk of heart disease, such as angina or a heart attack, and also of stroke. The large blood vessels that supply blood, for example to the legs, can also be affected (peripheral vascular disease) so that the lower legs may not get as much blood supply as needed. This can lead to problems such as severe pain in the calves when walking, or to leg or foot ulcers.

How can complications in large vessels be prevented and treated?

Again, tight control of blood glucose helps decrease the risk. The risk can also be decreased by not eating a diet that is very high in cholesterol and other fats or by not starting smoking. This also helps to keep your weight down, which in turn decreases the risk of developing high blood pressure. Regular exercise also decreases the risk. NICE recommends that children with diabetes have their blood pressure checked every year from the age of 12. High blood pressure and high cholesterol levels can be treated with oral medication, heart disease with medication and surgery.

Musculoskeletal complications

The musculoskeletal system is made up of the bones of the skeleton, muscles, and connective tissues such as tendons and ligaments. Connective tissue is made up of a substance called collagen. In diabetes, high blood glucose levels lead to glucose joining with the collagen to make the connective tissues stiff. This can lead to problems with the joints. One such problem is called 'limited joint mobility' (LJM). The joints of the hands and wrists are most often affected; for example, with LJM it may not be possible to put your hands together as if in prayer as the fingers stay bent. LJM is very closely associated with the small-vessels complications of diabetes. Other musculoskeletal conditions that are more likely in diabetes include carpal tunnel syndrome and frozen shoulder. The treatment for some musculoskeletal conditions includes anti-inflammatory painkillers, physiotherapy and steroid injections into the joint to reduce inflammation (these injections may increase blood glucose levels for 24 hours). Occasionally surgery may be needed.

Breast complications

It is rare to get complications in the breasts (diabetic mastopathy), and they tend not to occur until middle age. The tissue within the breast can become very hard and tough, sometimes with hard lumps. These lumps do not mean breast cancer. Every woman should regularly examine her breasts for lumps and any breast lumps should be examined as soon as possible by your doctor, so that breast cancer can be excluded.

Finally, remember that this chapter is not meant to scare you or to make you think that all these complications occur unless the diabetes is controlled, but to inform you. Without this knowledge you might not attend all your child's regular screening tests, which are very important. Good glucose control has been proven in many studies to decrease the risk of developing complications. Your child will not *definitely* get complications just because he has diabetes, and if any of them do develop, they won't *definitely* be in the most serious forms. With modern diabetic treatments, screening programmes, and treatments for complications in both their early and late stages, complications in their most severe forms may become increasingly less common.

Conditions associated with diabetes

Diabetes is an autoimmune disease, a condition in which the body attacks itself. If you have one autoimmune condition you are more likely to develop a second one. Therefore, people with diabetes are regularly screened for other autoimmune conditions, described below. Diabetes is also associated with various skin conditions and infections. Infections can be related to the diabetes and high blood glucose levels themselves or to the long-term complications of diabetes.

Autoimmune conditions

Hypothyroidism

The thyroid gland is found in the front of the neck and produces thyroid hormone, which has many functions in the body. For example, thyroid hormones affect the body's metabolic rate, development and growth. If you develop autoantibodies to the production of thyroid hormone, levels of thyroid hormone become low (hypothyroidism).

Symptoms
- there may be no symptoms;
- swelling in the neck – a goitre;
- tiredness and being lethargic;
- weight gain or a difficulty in losing weight (despite not eating more than usual, due to a decreased metabolic rate);
- mood changes such as depression;
- intolerance of cold;
- dry thin hair and dry skin;
- irregular or absent periods;

- more regular symptoms of hypoglycaemia, and you may not need very much insulin (due to the decreased metabolic rate).

How is hypothyroidism diagnosed and treated? Hypothyroidism is diagnosed by testing for thyroid hormones using a blood test. The National Institute for Health and Clinical Excellence (NICE) currently recommends screening for hypothyroidism at the time that diabetes is diagnosed, and then once a year. Hypothyroidism is treated by taking oral medicines which simply replace the amount of thyroid hormone needed.

Coeliac disease

In coeliac disease, the body attacks the small intestine. These attacks are triggered by a substance in wheat, barley and rye called gluten. The small intestine is where nutrients are absorbed from food, and so if it is damaged it can cause problems. Coeliac disease affects between 1 and 3 per cent of the population, but is ten times commoner if you have diabetes.

Symptoms
Symptoms commonly occur when cereals are introduced into the diet but can occur at any age.

- Not putting on weight as you should when growing (failure to thrive);
- poor appetite;
- bloating;
- tummy pain;
- diarrhoea;
- very light coloured and strong smelling stools;
- the muscles of the legs and buttocks may become very thin;
- with coeliac disease and diabetes, as food is not absorbed as it should be you may have more episodes of hypoglycaemia and not need very much insulin.

How is coeliac disease diagnosed and treated? Coeliac disease is diagnosed with blood tests to check for the autoantibodies that cause the condition. NICE currently recommends screening for coeliac disease with blood tests at the time that diabetes is diagnosed, and then every three years afterwards.

Coeliac disease is treated with a gluten-free diet – a diet free of anything containing wheat, barley or rye. On a gluten-free diet, the damage to the intestine is reversed. You may also need vitamin supplements. There are lots of gluten-free foods such as breads and pastas currently available.

Infections

Infections in diabetes can be both due to the condition itself and its long-term complications. White blood cells in the blood are part of the body's immune system and fight infections. When blood glucose levels are above 14 or 15 mmol/l, these white blood cells do not work as well as they should, increasing your risk of developing an infection.

Urine and bladder infections (urinary tract infections, UTIs) are very common in diabetes. This is due to both the decreased efficiency of the white blood cells but also due to the fact that bacteria need glucose to live and the urine in people with diabetics often contains glucose. Symptoms of urinary tract infections include fevers, tummy pain, urinating more frequently than normal or bedwetting, pain when urinating, strong or smelly urine and vomiting. They are treated with antibiotics. If your child has a urinary tract infection before the age of 5 years old, he will have further investigations to check the structure of the kidneys and bladder. These investigations start with an ultrasound scan, though other tests may be required.

Thrush is also more common in diabetes. Thrush is an infection with a fungus that often occurs in the genitals; the fungi are attracted to the high glucose levels. It is very common in girls and causes itching and burning in the vagina and skin of the genitals and a thick creamy whitish coloured discharge. Fungal infections can occur in boys under the foreskin, though fungal infections in boys are rarer than in girls. They are treated with either oral medication and/or creams to the affected area.

Infection is also more common in an area affected by diabetic neuropathy. For example, if you stand on something but do not have very good sensation in your feet, you may not be aware of the injury and won't clean the area appropriately. This, combined with the decreased functioning of the white blood cells at high blood glucose levels, increases the risk of developing an infection. An infection involving the skin and soft tissues is called cellulitis and is treated with antibiotics.

It is often thought that wounds or cuts heal more slowly in those with diabetes, again increasing the risk of infection. In children this may not be the case as they are unlikely to have developed problems with circulation to the feet and lower legs, so healing should be at the same speed as those without diabetes.

Skin conditions

It is common to get very itchy skin when blood glucose levels are high; this is because water is lost in the urine as well as glucose. This means that your skin gets dry, which makes it itchy.

Vitiligo is an autoimmune condition of the skin in which patches of skin lose their colour (pigmentation) and so develop patches of very white skin. Treatments include steroid creams and wearing high-factor suncream over the white patches to prevent them burning. A type of tattooing can be used so the areas match the rest of the skin.

A rare skin condition called necrobiosis lipoidica diabeticorum (NLD) can develop in the 30s and 40s, involving a rash of reddish brown patches. Currently the reason for developing this condition is not known, but it may be an autoimmune condition. A reddish-brown rash appears on the lower legs. Unfortunately, currently there is not a good treatment for NLD, though steroid creams and light therapy can be used.

People with type 2 diabetes may develop a skin condition called acanthosis nigricans. In this condition the skin in certain areas, such as the groin and armpits, becomes darker and thicker; it is often described as 'velvety'. This condition generally affects those who are overweight, and losing weight can improve the appearance of the skin.

9

Diabetes and infants, toddlers and primary-school-age children

Infants, toddlers and primary-school-age children represent a large age group, from very early childhood to about 11 years old, and issues differ depending on the age of the child. Some of the topics discussed, such as what teachers at school should be told or how diabetes should be managed during a sleepover, will also be relevant for older children in secondary school. You may have a situation that is not covered in this chapter, so as always, please refer to your diabetes team for further advice.

The management of diabetes in young children of different ages

The relationship between you, your child, his diabetes and its management depend on the age and maturity of your child. Very young children, such as those under two, are completely reliant on you for the management of their diabetes. Around the age of two, you may encounter the 'terrible twos', a time during which your child learns to say no, and may exert his own will as opposed to simply obeying you. As your child gets older he becomes inherently less self-centred and begins to develop an understanding of other people and the world. When he starts nursery and primary school he begins to make friends. Making friends is difficult and children are, often unintentionally, cruel. They notice when people are 'different'. It may be that your child feels different because of his diabetes, and this may be picked up on by school friends.

During all these stages, your child's development should not be affected by his diabetes, and he should be able to do the same things as his peers. His diabetes needs to be managed, but it should not stop him doing what he wants.

Issues that arise in very young children are often around injections and blood glucose monitoring. These can be painful and your child may find them difficult, perhaps especially difficult as they come from you, the person to whom he comes for protection and comfort. He may make you feel guilty and say hurtful things, perhaps unintentionally. Many parents may feel guilty that they are doing something that may make their child cry or be upset. Try to remember that you are aiming to help him, not harm him. The short-term pain and upset needs to be set against the benefits of having long-term good control of their diabetes. Be as matter of fact and calm as you can, as children respond to your own upset and fear. Even if your child is very young, speak in a calm voice and explain why you are doing the test.

Young children are not good verbal communicators. They may not be able to tell you that they are feeling hungry, thirsty or unwell. They may not be able to explain their symptoms of hypoglycaemia, which may then manifest as irritability, being whiny, clingy or in a temper tantrum. Maybe a temper tantrum means that you should be giving your child something to eat. However, if you do this every time, your child may learn that behaving badly means he gets food and so may act that way when not hypoglycaemic! The only way to know the difference between behaviour changes related to hypoglycaemia and the normal behaviour and mood changes of a child is with regular blood glucose testing.

Young children may perceive their diabetes, and the tests and injections it involves, as a punishment. They may think that they have done something wrong, or ask the age-old question 'why me'? They may feel frustrated and may want to be the same as everyone else. The younger your child, the more difficult he finds it to express these feelings, which may manifest as a refusal or stubbornness around injection time, or around what he is going to eat. Children with diabetes may develop problems with anxiety or depression; your diabetes team should be able to offer counselling or sessions with a psychologist.

As your child gets older he will be able to take more control over his injections and treatment. The average 8-year-old can perform his daily injections. However, even younger children can help get the equipment together for injections, or can place their hand on top of yours while giving an injection. Young children are often fascinated by how the body works, and you should try and explain as much as possible about their diabetes. For example, after a hypoglycaemic episode you could talk to your child about possible causes and why he felt unwell. It may well be that he does not understand everything first time; explanations may have to be repeated at the age-appropriate level on multiple occasions and lots of questions asked.

The most important thing is to keep talking. You and your child cannot hide from the fact that he has diabetes. It affects every aspect of his life, every day. Even a very young child can understand something about diabetes, or injections or tests. Try and explain to him why you are doing things. When you think he is old enough to have developed some understanding, you could try asking him questions about what you are doing and why you are doing it. With time, you can start asking his opinion about what treatment or tests should be carried out. In this way your child gradually gains more responsibility for looking after his diabetes. This process is very slow and gradual. It may not be complete for many years into adolescence, and as parents you still retain some responsibility, but it is important to at least start talking to your child as early as possible. Of course, relinquishing this control can be very difficult, but it is an important part of growing up. The child psychologist, counsellor and nurses on your diabetes team may be able to help you talk to your child and give you hints and tips on explaining diabetes to children and how to get them to take some responsibility for their own care.

Nursery and school

Teachers need to be aware that your child has diabetes. They need to know what treatment needs to be given in the day and what to do in emergencies. The organization Diabetes UK has information leaflets for teachers (see Useful Addresses). Depending on the age of your child, he may require help with his injections; for example, a nursery-age child needs significantly more help than a 10-year-old.

The diabetes specialist nurse on your team may be able to visit the school with you. You need to arrange a meeting with the school nurse and your child's form teacher. If your child has many different teachers (as occurs in secondary school) then all the teachers should be made aware of the child's condition. However, it may be more appropriate to appoint one teacher, such as the form teacher, to take the most responsibility for your child's management during the day.

At the meeting, you or your diabetes nurse could explain a little about what diabetes is, or give some written information. You need to show the teacher how to test a blood glucose level and give an injection. The teacher needs to tell you about the daily timetable and together you can make a management plan. For example, you need to know when lunchtime is and see the school menu so you and your child can decide what to eat and when alternative choices (even if it is sometimes just bread and butter) should be offered. It may be possible to make snack time the same time as break times in the school day. If this is not possible then some provision must be made so that your child can get appropriate snacks when needed. This may mean that you bring in a supply of snacks such as cereal bars or fruit and leave them in the school office or teacher's desk for your child to get when they are needed.

A common misconception is that people with diabetes must not eat sugar. This is not the case. Sugars are part of a healthy diet and during a hypoglycaemic episode sugar must be given. It is important that the teachers understand what hypoglycaemia is, its symptoms and how it should be treated. Sometimes the symptoms may be very vague, such as a lack of concentration. They must be aware that this is a situation that cannot wait until the end of class so that the hypoglycaemia does not worsen. You should leave a supply of glucose tablets or other sweet foods for such situations. Your child could either carry them around in her school bag or in her desk, or it may be more appropriate for the teacher to keep them in his or her desk. Inform teachers that after a hypoglycaemic attack the child may need another, longer-lasting snack such as a sandwich.

Your child needs to eat at approximately the same time each day, so if there is more than one sitting for lunch he needs to be in the same sitting each day. If you have the weekly timetable of the school menu and daily activities you can plan the insulin doses at home to tell the teacher. If your child is very young a teacher will have to give the injections – you or your diabetes nurse can show them how. Older children may be able to give their injections themselves, generally under supervision. The equipment needs to be stored in a safe and appropriate place where it cannot be accessed by other children. Many children will not want to have their injections in front of their friends. Injections generally have to be given before mealtimes. It may be appropriate that your child is excused from class for 10 minutes, half an hour before lunchtime to get his injection from the school nurse.

The requirements around physical activity and exercise should be explained. Diabetes is not a reason not to do exercise. Before or during a physical activity, the teacher should offer an extra snack or juice to prevent hypoglycaemia. Your child must have permission to eat at times when other children may be forbidden, such as during lessons, to prevent or treat hypoglycaemia.

School day trips should be treated as school days; your child and her teacher simply need to take their supplies of injection equipment, insulin and snacks as appropriate. With children, as at home, there is a balance to be struck at school between caring for their diabetes and letting them get on with their lives. It is important that children do not feel different or watched all the time. A care plan can be drawn up between you, your child, the diabetes team and the school as to how much responsibility the child should take and also his general daily management. Emergency plans can also be made. If, at any time, the teacher feels that a situation is escalating or he simply cannot manage he should ask for help or call the emergency services.

In secondary school, many children are able to give themselves injections and monitor their blood glucose if needed. However, the teachers still need to be informed of their condition and its management as above so that they are aware of the action required in an emergency and so your child can eat and access snacks etc. as required. As a parent you have a responsibility to inform the school as they take responsibility for your child during school hours.

Babysitters, grandparents, friend's parents

Anybody that, at some time, has responsibility for your child needs to be aware that he has diabetes and what, if any, treatment is needed, and what to do in an emergency. These people may include babysitters, nannies, grandparents, aunts and uncles and the parents of your child's friends, for example if they go over to play. The information given should be similar to that given to teachers, as described above. How much you need to explain depends on how long they look after your child. For example, if they are looking after your child for a couple of hours in the afternoon they may not need to know how to give an injection etc., but still need to know the importance of giving a snack or what to do in the event of hypoglycaemia. If possible, write down the information, as people find it a lot easier if they have a crib sheet they can look at if needed. If possible, leave a contact number for yourselves so you can be contacted in an emergency.

Telling friends

As much as your child may not want to be different from her friends, it is important that her friends know that she has diabetes. This explains why she may be treated differently in class, such as being allowed to eat. Your child will also spend time outside school with friends so it is important that they are aware of emergencies such as hypoglycaemia and what action needs to be taken. Depending on the age of the friends this can be simplified to something like giving sweets (which, for example, your child may always have in her bag) and getting help. Children are naturally very curious, so when they ask why your child is having an injection, be honest!

Birthday parties

Birthday parties are an important part of a child's social life. They involve special food and treats, presents and generally lots of activity, running around etc. Your child will be able to take part in everything. If you never let him have treats then they will become something that he may crave or sneak without your knowledge. Parties are special occasions and it is all right to let him eat sugar occasionally. Generally the sweets and junk food at a party are after a more substantial offering such as sandwiches and so make up part of a meal.

You could give an extra unit or so of insulin to counteract the sugar in birthday cake or sweets. As ever, though, this has to be weighed up against the level of activity at the party. If you know the party is going to be very active, such as a bouncy castle and soft-play party, you may not need the extra insulin as the glucose is used up in the activities. If, however, you know the party is going to be sedentary, such as an arts and crafts party, the extra insulin may be needed.

Treats are special occasions. If you find that your child is invited to birthday parties every weekend, and is being offered cake and sweets at each event, these foods are no longer treats but a part of the regular diet. In this scenario you may decide not to allow your child to eat sweets or may limit her to a small piece of cake. A hidden source of sugar is within fizzy drinks. You could provide a can of a 'diet' alternative, made with artificial sweeteners, for your child as these will not affect the blood sugar. Finally, test the blood glucose level when you get home from the party and record the level and the day's activity in your diary; this will help guide you as to the best course of action at the next birthday party.

Sleepovers and camps

During sleepovers children tend to stay up later than usual, playing games and may have a 'midnight feast', often of sweet foods. If your child is having a guest to stay you may want to offer an extra healthy late night snack to decrease the risk of hypoglycaemia. If your child is going to stay at a friend's house you need to tell the friend's parents about mealtimes and the extra snack, injections, hypoglycaemia etc. It may be easier to write down a timetable of food and injections so they have something to refer to. The same applies to going away on camp, or overnight school trips. You will have to pack supplies of insulin and equipment and supply the relevant information. You may feel anxious about someone else looking after your child's diabetes but this is not a reason not to let your child experience a good social life. Again, supplying a contact number will ease both your anxieties and those of the people looking after your child.

10

For teenagers: diabetes during puberty and adolescence

Puberty is a time of great change. In medical terms, adolescence is the stage of development between childhood and adulthood. Puberty relates to the time in which you become physically sexually mature and able to reproduce. One could say that puberty refers to the hormonal and chemical changes in the body that result in growth spurts and the maturation of sexual organs. Adolescence is a term that encompasses not just the physical changes but also the psychological and social changes of the teenage years.

Adolescence is a difficult time. Biologically, your body goes through many changes, some of which you may consider embarrassing or difficult to get used to. The surges of hormones may affect your mood. Psychologically, it is the time in which you move from being entirely dependent on your parents, as you were when you were a child, to being an independent adult. This change is difficult not just for you, but also for your parents, who may find it difficult to release their control. During this time, most people begin to think about their future and what kind of a person they want to be. It is a time of exploration of different ideas and experiences, when new relationships form and your sexuality develops. Each of these aspects can be confusing and take time to accept. This is no different whether or not you have diabetes. You may develop symptoms of anxiety or depression, and your diabetes team should be able to offer counselling or sessions with a psychologist.

If you do have diabetes there can be added complications and issues. Adolescence is the time of transition from your parents managing your diabetes treatment, to you taking control. As with all aspects of adolescence, your parents may find this difficult to accept. You may feel they are nagging you, continually asking you if you have taken your insulin and watching what you eat. It is very common for families to get into arguments around this issue: the parents feel they are trying to do what is best, and the children that the parents are interfering. As with most conflict, the best way to resolve the situation is to talk to each other. You could explain to your parents that you understand that they are only asking you these questions as they are concerned and looking out for your best interests, but that you are managing to cope alone. Reassuring them that you will ask for help when you need it may help them take a step back and stop pressurizing you. Alternatively, you may feel that your parents are pushing you to take too much responsibility. Again, talk to them, explain how you feel, that you are not ready to take on all the responsibility or that you are not sure how best to manage your diabetes. In this way, perhaps you could organize a gradual shift where they help you as much as needed while at the same time gradually increasing your involvement in your care.

Puberty is a time in which you will grow taller. You may have a growth spurt where you grow a lot in a short period of time, but even outside a growth spurt you will be growing. Growth is stimulated by the production of growth hormone in the brain. Growth hormone is one of the hormones that can also act to increase blood glucose levels. Therefore, during puberty, even if you do not change your diet or level of activity, you need more insulin than before to control your blood glucose levels. Once you have stopped growing, you will find that your insulin requirements fall again as they do not have to compensate for the extra growth hormone. For more information on insulin requirements in puberty, please refer to Chapter 5, 'Treatment of diabetes'.

Adolescence is also a time in which you start to think about relationships and sex. You may start going out a lot with your friends or staying up very late at night. You may start drinking alcohol or smoking or be very concerned about your weight. These topics are discussed in this chapter. You are able to do everything that your friends and peers do, but you simply have to take care of your diabetes at the same time. You may think that there is no point in caring about your diabetes, that you will develop complications anyway, or you may want to rebel against the strict diabetes control that you feel your parents inflicted upon you. Remember, though: having diabetes does not mean that you will definitely develop complications or that you cannot do something that you want to; you just have to look after yourself. With good control, you will find that diabetes is simply another part of your everyday life.

Diabetes and your body weight

Your body changes significantly during puberty. You grow taller, you develop hair in new places, if you are a girl your breasts develop and you start your periods, while if you are a boy your genitals will change and your voice drop. Concerns about keeping your body weight under control are very common.

While growing, you need to eat more than previously as your body needs the extra fuel. However, once you stop growing, if you continue to eat more than your body needs you will put on weight – a common reason for people to gain weight in adolescence. The extra food can be in any form. It is not simply that if you eat extra chocolate you put on weight – even if you are eating more than you need of something that is good for you, like a baked potato, if you are eating more calories than your body needs, it stores the extra food as fat and you gain weight. However, healthy foods often contain fewer calories than junk food, and fill you up for longer, so you are less likely to eat more than necessary.

If you have diabetes, it can be very difficult to lose any extra weight. You cannot simply dramatically reduce the amount you eat or ignore the warning symptoms of hypoglycaemia. Once you have taken your insulin, you need to eat. However, you can lose weight by changing what it is that you eat.

If your HbA1c and therefore your blood glucose levels are continually high, you lose glucose in your urine; your cells still need the same amount of glucose but you have to eat more to compensate for the amount of glucose lost in the urine. Therefore having a high HbA1c can make you lose weight. However, this is a dangerous method of weight loss. It puts you at a higher risk of developing severe hyperglycaemia and ketoacidosis, and increases your risk of long-term complications. Many teenagers may try to use this method to help them lose weight but it does have potentially dangerous consequences. Speak to your diabetes team or try the tips below to help you lose weight without resorting to this dangerous method. If you have had high blood glucose levels for a while you need initially to take more insulin than normal as the body has become insulin resistant. When you start taking insulin again, the cells take up the extra glucose in the blood and initially you put on weight. However, your body quickly becomes sensitive to insulin again, and this combined with decreasing your food intake helps you lose weight.

Discuss your weight with your dietician and the diabetes team. You want to start slowly reducing the amount of food you eat each day as you begin to stop growing. If you are reducing the amount of food you eat, you also need to reduce the amount of insulin that you take, in order to prevent hypoglycaemic attacks. You need to look at what you eat and try and make your diet as healthy as possible, for example by not eating processed foods and instead eating lots of fruit and vegetables. You should not miss meals as that will increase the risk of hypoglycaemia. Instead regularly eat foods that release energy slowly to stop you getting hungry in between meals. Weight loss should be slow and gradual – even losing about a pound or half a kilo per week adds up to about 25 kg or nearly four stone in a year! Get your parents and family involved. It is much easier for you to stick to a healthy diet if people around you are also eating healthily. You are much less likely to eat unhealthy food if it is not in the house! For more information on a healthy diet, see Chapter 6, 'Diet and staying well'.

If you do become hypoglycaemic, either because you have not eaten enough or because the insulin dose is too high, you must not ignore the symptoms. Test your blood glucose to check that you truly are hypoglycaemic and eat as appropriate; you need to eat something sweet that you may not have been allowing yourself in your diet but it is important to reverse the hypoglycaemia. Do not overeat, though – eat a little, wait about 10 to 15 minutes and then eat a bit more if necessary.

Eating disorders often start in adolescence. The prevalence of eating disorders in older teenagers has been quoted as between 1 and 5 per cent, and they are more common in girls than in boys. The term eating disorders covers both anorexia nervosa and bulimia nervosa. In anorexia, there is significant weight loss and people's view of their own body weight is distorted; they feel that they are fat when others believe they are very thin, and have a powerful fear of becoming overweight. As a consequence, they hugely restrict what they eat, and the amount of calories, and may also partake in a lot of exercise in an attempt to lose weight. Bulimia is also characterized by a distorted view of body weight; instead of restricting calorie intake, there is binge eating followed by purging, either by vomiting or use of laxatives in an attempt to control weight. Bulimia and anorexia can exist together.

People with diabetes can be affected by eating disorders. However, their bodies cannot cope as well as those without diabetes with vomiting, significantly decreased calorie intake or excessive exercise. Not using insulin as a method of losing weight increases the risk of developing ketoacidosis and long-term diabetic complications. This is sometimes called 'diabulimia'. If you feel that you need help, please contact your doctors. You may need input from both your diabetic team as well as the psychological and/or the psychiatric eating disorders team.

Periods, sex and fertility

When you start having periods they are often irregular for the first year or so. Having poor blood glucose control and a high HbA1c increases the risk of your periods staying irregular. You may notice that your blood glucose levels increase slightly just before your period so you may need more insulin. Not everyone has this pattern. In your diabetes diary you could also write down where in your menstrual cycle you think you are so that you can see if any patterns develop.

The legal age of consent in the United Kingdom is 16 years of age. There is no difference in sexual desire or the ability to have sex in teenagers with diabetes to those without. You may find that you need to eat extra snacks or decrease the amount of insulin you use when you are having sex as it is exercise. Girls may find that if their blood glucose levels are high they get very dry and itchy genitals that may make sexual intercourse painful, but this can generally be relieved with a lubricant. One of the long-term complications of diabetes may be problems with erections, but this should not be a regular problem in teenage boys (though it does occur occasionally in most people, generally due to anxiety).

If you want to prevent pregnancy you need to use contraception. Condoms are the only form of contraception that prevents the risk of both pregnancy and of getting a sexually transmitted disease, and they are available free of charge at family planning clinics. Even if you are under 16, speak to your GP about the different kinds of contraception as they may be able to give you a prescription for the contraceptive that is most appropriate. As long as certain conditions are met, your GP will not have to inform your parents that you have requested contraception.

A common concern in girls is how diabetes may affect their ability to get pregnant. As long as your diabetes control is good, your fertility should not be affected. If you are thinking about becoming pregnant then you should inform your diabetes team. There are risks related to diabetes and pregnancy including a higher risk of having a very large baby, congenital malformations and for the baby to be hypoglycaemic after birth. These risks are decreased with good control of your blood glucose before and during your pregnancy. You will be closely monitored by your diabetic and obstetric team. The fact that you have diabetes does not necessarily mean that your child will become diabetic.

Diabetes and alcohol

The legal age at which you can buy alcohol in the United Kingdom is 18, though many younger teenagers drink alcohol. When you drink alcohol it is broken down in the liver. While the liver is busy dealing with the alcohol it cannot produce glucose from its glycogen stores when needed, so drinking lots of alcohol increases the risk of hypoglycaemia. This hypoglycaemia occurs even in people without diabetes and can occur many hours after drinking, even into the next day, as it takes the liver a long time to break down alcohol (one hour for every unit of alcohol). Alcohol affects the brain: initially it might make you feel good, but it also affects your ability to respond to situations and therefore your ability to look after your diabetes.

If you have diabetes you may notice that your blood sugar rises just after a drink, due to the carbohydrate or sugar content of the alcohol. You are then at risk of hypoglycaemia, especially if you have also been doing extra exercise, such as when clubbing. You can prevent this by eating an extra snack containing carbohydrates both before and after drinking and monitor your blood glucose regularly. Try not to oversleep as you may become hypoglycaemic in the morning from the effects of sugar – instead, set an alarm, test your blood sugar, eat if appropriate and then go back to sleep! Make sure that your friends know that you are diabetic, otherwise they may just assume that you are drunk as opposed to hypoglycaemic if you are diabetic.

No one can tell you how much you are 'allowed' to drink. You have to make your own decisions, but being aware and able to prepare for the consequences of drinking and its potential effects on your blood glucose enables you to make an informed decision.

Diabetes and smoking

The legal age at which you can buy cigarettes in the United Kingdom is now 18, though many teenagers younger than this start smoking. Put simply, smoking is bad for you. It increases your risk of developing among other things lung disease, heart disease and cancer. Some of the long-term complications of diabetes include having a heart attack or a stroke. If you smoke as well as have diabetes, the risk of your developing one of these conditions is significantly increased. The nicotine in cigarettes can also increase insulin resistance, so your diabetes may become more difficult to control.

People who smoke become addicted to the nicotine in cigarettes so it is very difficult to give up. It is far easier not to start smoking than to give it up. If you have started smoking, then your doctor may be able to help you give up by prescribing you nicotine replacement therapy.

Diabetes and recreational drug use

Recreational drugs are illegal, no matter how old you are. They are illegal because they are dangerous and often addictive. They affect the brain and while they may make you feel a certain way that you may enjoy, they also affect your decision-making skills so you may neglect your diabetes. For example, cannabis may make you very hungry so you may eat excessively resulting in hyperglycaemia; ecstasy or speed may suppress your appetite, increasing the risk of developing hypoglycaemia.

School stresses

School can be stressful for a number of reasons, from difficulties with friends, exam stresses and competitive sports. Each of these stresses affects your insulin requirements.

All your teachers, including your PE teachers, should be aware that you have diabetes. You may have to adjust your insulin requirements on the days that you have PE or a sports competition and may have to eat an extra snack before starting the exercise. Having diabetes does not mean that you are unable to compete in sports, even at a very high level. You will have to adjust your diabetes management accordingly.

Hypoglycaemia makes it difficult to concentrate, even in the few hours after a hypoglycaemic attack when your blood glucose levels may be back to normal. Therefore you should aim for normal blood glucose levels so you can concentrate to the best of your ability during lessons. This is especially important before and during exams. Have something extra to eat before an exam and take a snack into the exam hall. Some people prefer to eat extra, even if it makes them slightly hyperglycaemic, to prevent hypoglycaemia. Schools often have a no-eating policy during exams, but as long as they are aware that you have diabetes this rule should not apply to you. If you feel unwell during an exam you should take your blood glucose level and show your teacher. If you do not perform as well as you think you should during an exam and you think you have got a low grade because you were hypoglycaemic, this evidence of low blood glucose and a doctor's letter may lead to the exam board adjusting your marks.

The body reacts to any form of stress by secreting adrenaline.

Adrenaline is one of the hormones that acts to bring up blood glucose levels. During times of stress your blood sugar levels rise and you need more insulin to compensate. Stress can be physical such as an illness, or emotional, such as anxiety about exams. Having problems at home with your siblings or parents, having an argument with your friends, or even watching a scary film can be stressful and may affect your blood glucose. We should all try and decrease the level of stress in our lives, whether or not we have diabetes. Stress is natural and inevitable: the adrenaline produced during stress gives us the ability to cope with stressful situations. In diabetes, your management may have to be adjusted accordingly.

Going out with friends

As you gain independence from your parents, your social life may become more important. You may stay out late or up all night with your friends, or may spend time clubbing or dancing at parties. This affects your diabetes control – after all, dancing is exercise! If you are staying up late or all night, eat regularly throughout the night, at least every five hours as you would in the daytime. Do not give yourself your night-time insulin at your normal time but use a short-acting insulin before these extra meals to control your blood glucose. Adjust the dosage of insulin according to how much you eat and how much exercise such as dancing you think you will do.

Having a lie-in

Having a late night out is often followed by a long lie-in the next day. How this affects your diabetes depends on what you did and how much insulin you took during the previous evening. For example, if you drank a lot of alcohol you are at risk of hypoglycaemia and so should set your alarm to check your blood sugar. If, however, you have not drunk alcohol and simply stayed up late then you could take your night-time insulin dose when you go to bed, even if it is 3 a.m. You will probably still sleep the same amount of time as if you had gone to bed earlier at your normal time. Your night-time dose works as normal, you have just given it later, and instead of working from 10 p.m. to 7 a.m., it will work from 3 a.m. to midday.

If you wake up late and then shift your mealtimes later, then you can use your normal insulin dose for breakfast. You have to shift the time of taking your insulin according to when you eat your meals. If you go to bed very late but intend to get up early, or at your normal time, you need to adjust your night-time insulin dose. You need to decrease the dose to compensate for the shorter period of time that you are asleep; you then take your breakfast dose as normal.

Travelling

When travelling you need to take all your diabetes supplies with you. Take much more insulin than you think you need, in case some gets damaged or you need to take extra. You should obtain travel insurance or a European Health Insurance Card if you are travelling within the European Union, and take documentation that says you are a diabetic as you may need to explain to airport security or staff why you are carrying medication that includes needles. Carry all your medication in your hand luggage for use on the plane or in case your luggage gets lost or is exposed to freezing temperatures in the hold. Try not to expose your insulin to too hot or cold temperatures. If you take copies of your prescriptions a doctor may prescribe you more insulin wherever you are if your supply becomes unusable. Remember to check the concentration of the insulin supplied, as it may be different to what you are used to.

It is very common to develop diarrhoea and/or vomiting while travelling, 'traveller's tummy'. You can try and prevent this by only drinking clean water and avoiding undercooked food. If you do develop diarrhoea, try and keep yourself hydrated. You may need to drink oral rehydration solution and keep a close eye on your blood glucose levels.

You may need to adjust your insulin and food intake according to your level of activity on your holiday. For example, a holiday lying on a beach involves far less activity than hiking or skiing. Diving is the one sport that you may not be allowed to partake in; different diving schools have different regulations. It may be that you are allowed to dive as long as your diabetes control has been very good for at least a year and you have your doctor's permission. The reason for the strict rules around diving is that it is very difficult to respond to an emergency such as hypoglycaemia while deep underwater, and it is not always possible to rise to the surface very quickly without potentially causing other harmful conditions such as the 'bends'. If you are allowed to dive, eat an extra snack before diving to prevent hypoglycaemia, as diving is exercise, and make sure everyone on your dive is aware of your condition.

Driving and diabetes

You can start to learn to drive at 17 years old in the United Kingdom. You have to inform the Driving Vehicle Licensing Authority (DVLA) and your car insurance that you have diabetes. The DVLA then asks you to contact them if there are any changes in your condition that may affect your ability to drive, such as eyesight problems. The DVLA does not allow people with diabetes to have a licence to drive heavy goods or passenger-carrying vehicles such as a bus, though you can drive a taxi. Not telling your insurance company can invalidate your insurance if you do have an accident.

Hypoglycaemia while driving can be dangerous. Even if you do not have many symptoms, your reaction times may be slowed, which can increase the risk of having an accident. Therefore, you should not drive if you know you are hypoglycaemic. If you get symptoms of hypoglycaemia while you are driving, pull over, check your blood glucose if possible and eat something. You should have glucose tablets or snacks in your car for such occasions.

Choosing a job

Most jobs should pose no problems to you even if you have diabetes. Depending on the level of activity within the job you may have to adjust your insulin doses. For example, if you do a job that requires lots of physical activity such as being a builder, you need extra snacks or less insulin. Unfortunately you will not be able to work within the military services.

If there is a health question on a job application form you must declare that you have diabetes. As long as you have not been asked it is not a legal requirement to inform your colleagues that you have diabetes, though it is advisable so you can manage your condition openly. There may be a misconception that having diabetes means that you will be taking lots of time off work, but you can reassure your colleagues that this is not the case. You cannot be refused a job (apart from in the military, or as a bus driver) on the basis that you have diabetes. If you feel that you have been unfairly refused a job, or been sacked from a job because of your diabetes, you can appeal under the Disability Discrimination Act. Under the terms of the Act, it is illegal to discriminate against you because of your diabetes.

Money

You may be eligible for a grant if you go to college or university (a disabled student allowance). As with the Disability Discrimination Act, it is not saying that because you have diabetes you are disabled. Not everyone with diabetes is eligible for the grant, but everyone is eligible to apply.

Transfer to adult services

The transfer from the care of the paediatric diabetic team to the adult team can be a difficult time. After all, you will have got to know the members of your diabetic team very well, probably over years. You may have had a paediatric emergency card, which allowed you not to wait in A & E if you needed treatment, but to be seen straight away by the paediatric team. This will not occur once you are in adult services: in an emergency you always have to go to A & E. The adult team will consist of the people in similar jobs to the paediatric team. You will have a consultant who is a specialist in diabetes or endocrinology (hormones), diabetes specialist nurses and dieticians. The change between teams may be done gradually; in some areas the adult teams have age-specific clinics, in which case you would be placed in a young adults' clinic. The age at which the transfer occurs will depend on the service provision in your area; generally it occurs between the ages of 16 and 18.

11

Future developments

Research into diabetes is widespread, ongoing and often in the press. Research into the causes of diabetes aims to be able to prevent new cases from occurring and also to find a cure – if we know why something happens we are in a much better position to find out how to stop it. Research into treatments involves trying to find new ways of monitoring diabetes, preventing complications and delivering insulin; research into a cure aims to avoid the need for treatment altogether.

Research into the causes of diabetes focuses on trying to find out the exact process that leads to the development of diabetes. For example, if diabetes is solely an autoimmune disease then a treatment could be developed that interacts with the body's immune system to prevent the body from attacking itself and therefore prevents diabetes occurring.

Research into treatments includes new methods of delivering insulin and measuring blood glucose: for example, research into blood glucose meters that either involve extremely tiny needles that barely pierce the skin or do not even need needles at all. Other research is being carried out into a meter that is implanted just under the skin and can continuously measure blood glucose so you will always know what your blood glucose levels are. These meters could be set with an alarm to alert you if your blood glucose is getting too high or you are becoming hypoglycaemic.

A lot of research is being carried out into finding different ways of giving insulin that do not involve regular injections. Options being investigated include giving insulin as a nasal spray or inhalation (like an asthma pump). An oral tablet is also being investigated; any tablet has to withstand the acid environment of the stomach to prevent the insulin being broken down before it gets to the small intestine where it can be used.

Research into cures for diabetes includes gene therapy, stem-cell therapy and transplants. Gene therapy involves manipulating the genes of a cell to correct a genetic problem. Correctly functioning genes – in the case of diabetes this could be those that lead to the production of insulin – could be inserted into affected cells using modified (and therefore hopefully harmless) viruses to carry the genes into the cells.

The aim is that the cells would then start to produce insulin on their own and therefore the diabetes would be cured.

A stem cell is a cell that has the potential to become any kind of cell in the body, from a skin cell to a brain cell. Stem cells are found in developing embryos and in the umbilical cord that attaches the developing baby to its mother. Adult stem cells can be found in the bone marrow, though these are already more specialized and can only form any of the different blood cells. Once a stem cell has evolved into a certain type of cell it cannot change to become another type, so once it is a stomach-lining cell it cannot become a muscle cell. It may become possible to use stem cells to form new pancreatic cells that can then produce insulin. Stem therapy raises many ethical issues such as how stem cells are collected. For example, should scientists be allowed to collect stem cells from aborted foetuses?

Transplants involve taking organs or parts of organs from one person, matched genetically as closely as possible, and putting them in another person. In the case of diabetes, the transplant can be either of the whole pancreas, or the insulin-producing cells of the islets of Langerhans can be transplanted into the affected person's liver. The problem with transplants is that, unless you have an identical twin, no one has exactly the same genetic make-up and so your body recognizes that the transplant is 'foreign' and tries to reject it. In order to stop this process occurring, powerful drugs must be used that often have significant side effects.

Research takes time and you may read about new developments in the press that are many years away from being available to the public, as any treatment has to go through very rigorous testing to ensure that it is safe.

Useful addresses

UK and Ireland

Diabetes Careline
Macleod House
10 Parkway
London NW1 7AA
Tel.: 0845 120 2960 (9 a.m. to 5 p.m., Monday to Friday)

Part of Diabetes UK (see below), it provides support and information regarding diabetes by trained counsellors via its helpline.

Diabetes Federation of Ireland
76 Lower Gardiner Street
Dublin 2, Republic of Ireland
Tel.: 01 836 3022
Helpline: 1 850 909 909
Website: www.diabetesireland.ie
Email: info@diabetes.ie

Aims to represent people with diabetes in Ireland, provide information and support and encourage research.

Diabetes Insight
c/o Trefoil Solutions Ltd
15 Ravenhill Avenue
Knowle
Bristol BS3 5DU
Website: www.diabetes-insight.info

Seeks to provide information through online support groups and forums for people affected by diabetes.

Diabetes UK
Central Office, Macleod House
10 Parkway
London NW1 7AA
Tel.: 020 7424 1000
Website: www.diabetes.org.uk
Email: info@diabetes.org.uk

The largest diabetes charity in the UK, with regional offices around the country, Diabetes UK aims to improve the lives of people with diabetes, and their families and carers, by campaigning on their behalf, supplying information and funding research.

Food Standards Agency
(Healthy-eating division)
Website: www.eatwell.gov.uk

The Food Standards Agency seeks to protect public health with respect to food safety. Its healthy-eating division provides information on a healthy diet.

Insulin Dependent Diabetes Trust
PO Box 294
Northampton NN1 4XS
Tel.: 01604 622837
Website: www.iddtinternational.org
Email: enquiries@iddtinternational.org

Aims to raise general awareness about diabetes, and offers support to those affected, and to their families and carers.

Insulin Pumpers UK
Website: www.insulin-pumpers.org.uk

The UK division of the international society promoting the use of insulin pumps in the treatment of diabetes. Provides information and support for pump users.

Juvenile Diabetes Research Foundation
19 Angel Gate
City Road
London EC1V 2PT
Tel.: 020 7713 2030
Website: www.jdrf.org.uk
Email: info@jdrf.org.uk

The UK branch of the Juvenile Diabetes Research Foundation International (see below), providing information and support to children and adolescents with diabetes, and their families. Aims to promote research to find a cure and prevent diabetic complications.

NHS Direct
Tel.: 0845 46 47
Website: www.nhsdirect.nhs.uk

NHS Direct aims to give the general public access to information regarding their health. The phone number, open 24 hours a day, allows you to speak to a nurse adviser who can help you over the phone or recommend you to go to your doctor or local hospital as appropriate.

Overseas

American Diabetes Association
1701 North Beauregard Street
Alexandria
VA 22311
USA
Website: www.diabetes.org

A not-for-profit organization providing information on diabetes and support, and involved in research.

Children with Diabetes
5689 Chancery Place
Hamilton
OH 45011
USA
Website: www.childrenwithdiabetes.com

This organization, which possesses an excellent website, seeks to promote education regarding diabetes and its treatments, and gives support to children, adolescents, carers and families.

International Diabetes Federation
Avenue Emile De Mot 19
B-1000 Brussels
Belgium
Tel.: +32 2 5385511
Website: www.idf.org
Email: info@idf.org

An international organization aiming to promote the awareness of diabetes, good care, and research into a cure, and into prevention of the condition.

International Society for Paediatric and Adolescent Diabetes
c/o KIT, Kurfürstendamm 71
10709 Berlin
Germany
Tel.: +49 30 24603213
Website: www.ispad.org
Email: secretariat@ispad.org

An association catering specifically for children and adolescents with diabetes, and aiming to promote the best care possible for them.

Juvenile Diabetes Research Foundation International
120 Wall Street, 19th Floor
New York NY 1005-4001
USA
Website: www.jdrf.org
Email: info@jdrf.org

This international organization, of which the Juvenile Diabetes Research Foundation in the UK (see above) is a branch, promotes research into the condition.

National Diabetes Information Clearinghouse
1 Information Way
Bethesda
MD 20892-3560
USA
Tel.: 1-800-860-8747
Website: http://diabetes.niddk.nih.gov
Email: ndic@info.niddk.nih.gov

A service provided by an American agency, the National Institute of Diabetes and Digestive and Kidney Diseases, it aims to increase knowledge of diabetes among patients, their families and the general public. There are lots of resources on the website.

Index

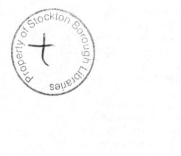